Dissertation Research & Writing for Construction Students

- User-friendly, easy-to-dip-into guide for all Built Environment students
- Takes the reader from the stage of choosing a topic to writing a well-structured dissertation
- Best case practice illustrated with numerous examples, case studies and references

Dissertation Research & Writing for Construction Students covers topic selection, research planning, data collection and methodology, as well as structuring and writing the dissertation – in fact, everything needed for a successful write-up.

A new section advising students on the use of the SPSS software package Statistical Analysis for Social Sciences will help readers make the best use of this tool. New examples and references ensure that this new edition of the bestselling construction dissertation guide is right up to speed with current practice.

This is the ideal resource for students involved in research in Construction Management, Building and Quantity Surveying.

Dr S. G. Naoum is a Senior Lecturer in the Department of Property, Surveying and Construction at London South Bank University. Before beginning his academic career he worked as a site engineer and project manager.

Dissertation Research & Writing for Construction Students

Third edition
Dr S. G. Naoum

Routledge
Taylor & Francis Group

LONDON AND NEW YORK

First edition published 1998
by Butterworth-Heinemann

This edition published 2013
by Routledge
2 Park Square, Milton Park, Abingdon, Oxon, OX14 4RN

Simultaneously published in the USA and Canada
by Routledge
711 Third Avenue, New York, NY 10017

Routledge is an imprint of the Taylor & Francis Group, an informa business

British Library Cataloguing in Publication Data
A catalogue record for this book is available from the British Library

Library of Congress Cataloging-in-Publication Data
Naoum, S. G. (Shamil G.)
Dissertation research and writing for construction students / Shamil
Naoum. — 3rd ed.
p. cm.
Includes bibliographical references and index.
1. Dissertations, Academic. 2. Technical writing. I. Title.
LB2369.N27 2012
808.02—dc23
2012006108

ISBN13: 978-0-415-53844-2 (pbk)

Typeset in Times New Roman by Prepress Projects Ltd, Perth, UK

To my mother, Rose

Contents

Preface

This book has grown out of my involvement in supervising BSc and MSc dissertations as well as my accumulated experience of teaching research methods to postgraduate students at London South Bank University. Over the years, I became convinced that construction students needed something akin to research methods lectures, in addition to tutoring, that could provide them with guidance on basic research techniques and how to write a dissertation. There have been an enormous number of textbooks which presented research design and methodologies but few, if any, are related to built environment studies.

This book approaches dissertation research and writing as a process, involving a sequence of learnable activities. Each activity prepares the student for the next step and some steps are best taken before others. I have divided the process of dissertation research into three parts, which are best carried out in the order presented.

Part I is 'preparing the ground'. It involves:

1. identifying the problem (including narrowing and clarifying the problem);
2. writing a proposal (including the aim, objectives, hypothesis and/or key research questions;
3. reviewing the literature (including critical appraisal of literature).

Part II is 'research design'. It involves:

4. approaches to data collection (deciding whether to use a survey or a case study);
5. techniques for data collection (deciding whether to use the post or go for interviews);
6. constructing and sampling the questionnaire.

Part III is 'analysis of the results' and producing the dissertation. It involves:

7. measurement of data;
8. analysis of data (including interpretation and discussion of results);
9. structuring and writing the whole dissertation;
10. dissertation supervision and assessment.

This book is aimed specifically at BSc and MSc students, who are embarking on research as part of their degree. It will provide students with a clear explanatory text which is supported by numerous examples illustrating good practice. Students of Built Environment subjects such as Construction Management, Facility Management, Building Surveying, Quantity Surveying and Civil Engineering will find this book of use. It will also be of use to those candidates requiring membership of the Chartered Institute of Building (CIOB) and anyone else involved in research work.

About the third edition

It has been very pleasing to receive the many complimentary and positive comments from reviewers and users of the first and second editions. These comments have been most appreciated and provided the encouragement for, the basis of, the third edition.

The third edition retains the same underlying theme, aims and approaches. It also carriers forward the same basic framework with the same sequencing and ordering of the chapters.

There is, however, a general review and update of material. The rationalisation of the text recognises the need for new sections such as 'examples of research road maps', 'further examples of writing a literature review', 'further examples of data analysis', 'the use of SPSS' and 'additional appendices'.

Acknowledgements

I wish to express my special thanks and appreciation to David Coles for his encouragement during the preparation of the first edition of this book.

I am also grateful to the following students for their permission to extract information from their dissertations: Miss H. Cooper, Mr S. Green, Mr B. Hemmings, Mr M. Howard, Mrs Z. Mulholland, Mr F. Rassam and Mr T. Whitworth.

I also wish to thank Longman Group Ltd, London, for permission to adapt appendices from their book *Statistical Tables for Biological, Agricultural, and Medical Research*, sixth edition (1974); to Pitman Publishing, for permission to adapt a table from their book, *Management and Organisational Behaviour*, fourth edition (1996); and to Unwin Hyman Publications, for permission to adapt a table from their book, *Quantity and Quality in Social Research* (1988). Last but not least my thanks go to my colleague D. Fong for his permission to use his SPSS lecture notes, which are exhibited in Appendix 5.

References to sources of information and material are given as accurately as possible throughout this book. Apologies are expressed if any acknowledgement has inadvertently not been recorded.

Finally, I wish to express my gratitude to the staff of Prepress Projects Ltd, who masterfully crafted the production of this book.

Dr Shamil Naoum
Department of Built Environment
London South Bank University

1 *Introduction*

This book provides a guide and learning support document in the preparation of a dissertation for honours undergraduate students and for students undertaking dissertations on taught Masters degrees. The book focuses specifically on built environment subjects with a special reference to the discipline areas of Construction, Project Management, Quantity Surveying, Building Surveying, Estate Management, Facility Management and others. However, as the book follows the interrelated process of conducting a research, it can also be useful to undergraduate and postgraduate students of various disciplines. It covers issues such as the selection of a dissertation topic, writing a proposal, conducting a literature review, selecting the research approach, devising research instruments, collecting information, analysing and presenting information and producing a well-written dissertation.

Rationale for conducting a dissertation

The rationale for including a dissertation as a major component of the BSc and MSc courses is that it provides for the development of intellectual skills of a kind that is not fully facilitated on the other components of the teaching course. The dissertation requirement accords with the educational philosophy of the BSc and MSc course in that it requires students to take responsibility for their own learning, specifying and defining the task, and defining the learning outcomes.

The aims and objectives of conducting a dissertation are therefore:

1 To provide the opportunity for students to undertake an independent piece of work of a demanding nature.
2 To enable students to investigate, in depth, a subject in which they have a particular interest and of their own selection.
3 To provide students with an opportunity to stretch their intellectual and technical skills.
4 To encourage students to develop new forms of analysis, conclusions and policies which may make an original contribution to the knowledge in the field of study concerned.

5   To encourage both clarity and depth of thought in that the project involves analysis of a problem in depth and the development of a logical sequence of ideas.

6   To provide students with an opportunity of learning how to acquire detailed information on a particular issue. It will involve them in the use of bibliographies, libraries and library reference systems. It will involve them in using primary sources of data such as a census, and it will involve the collection of new data through interviews, surveys and archival research.

7   To require the proper use, presentation and communication of data.

The meaning of research

The *Concise Oxford Dictionary* defines research as 'careful search or inquiry; endeavour to discover new or collate old facts etc. by scientific study of a subject; course of critical investigation' (Soanes and Stevenson, 2004). From this we can conclude that the word 'research' may be used interchangeably with 'inquiry', 'study' or 'investigation'. And yet something more is implied: the inquiry, study or investigation must be conducted in a careful, scientific and/or critical manner. Others have added to this list of adjectives 'methodical' and 'systematic'. It does not really matter which combination of words is chosen (systematic inquiry or critical investigation) so long as both words are kept clearly in mind.

In addition to a specific method of inquiry, a research project has to have an aim or objective. In general terms, the aim of all research is to expand knowledge. But we do not simply want a list of facts. A good piece of research will focus on certain aspects of a topic. It will seek to answer specific questions, solve a particular problem or test a hypothesis. The issue(s) to be addressed must be clearly stated at the outset in the objective(s) of research.

Purpose of the book

This book fulfils the need of the construction industry by providing students with a useful guide to undertake a piece of research. The construction industry is now developing a community with a new attitude to research. Although a number of texts are available on research design and methodology, there is little, if any, applied in construction. This book is specifically designed to assist:

1   Honours undergraduate students in Built Environment with specific emphasis on construction-related degree programmes;

2   MSc (taught Masters) students in Construction Management/Project Management-related subjects;

3   CIOB (member) new educational framework course programmes offered by universities, colleges of higher educational, correspondence courses, and so on;

4   CIOB (direct member) thesis route programme.

The book will also assist:

1   students of other related Built Environment disciplines, for example Building Surveying, Quantity Surveying, Architecture, Building Economics, Facility Management, Estate Management, and Commercial Management;
2   students in the social sciences and people concerned with social surveys.

Additionally, the book should provide a useful 'foundation' guide to students who are about to start an MPhil/PhD programme. However, it is not designed to provide a manual for PhD students, nor does it provide the type of analysis that a doctorate deserves.

Plan of the book

As mentioned earlier, this book will follow the interrelated stages of conducting a dissertation research. Figure 1.1 illustrates the research process stages with their corresponding chapters. This book is therefore composed of 10 chapters.

Chapter 1: Introduction

This chapter provides a general introduction to dissertation research and outlines the main aims and objectives of the book.

Chapter 2: Selecting a topic and writing the dissertation proposal

The choice of a dissertation topic usually comes from your interest in and value of a particular subject, which are usually interrelated. The interest and value will eventually be developed into a series of questions, which you will be keen to find answers to. Selecting a topic is discussed in the first part of the chapter. After selecting the subject of your dissertation, you need to formulate a proposal that should contain a rationale, research goals (aim, objectives, hypothesis or key questions), outline methodology and a programme of work. The extent and degree of details for the dissertation proposal are given in the second part of this chapter.

Chapter 3: Reviewing the literature

This activity will most likely be carried out throughout the whole research process but more extensively at the earlier stages of the research. It basically involves reading and critically appraising what other people have written about your subject area. The chapter also gives details on how to conduct a systematic literature search.

Figure 1.1 *Research process diagram.*

Chapter 4: Approaches to data collection

After deciding on the topic that you wish to study and having conducted an extensive literature search, you will be in a position to design your research. Designing the research involves the following activities:

1 Deciding on the type of data that has to be collected (quantitative or qualitative data). This chapter provides further description of these terms.
2 Confirm the method of data collection (i.e. should you conduct a survey or a case study). The chapter describes each of these methods in great detail.
3 Deciding on the techniques for data collection (i.e. should you gather the data by interviews, by telephone or by postal questionnaire?).
4 Designing your sample. The research design should tell you how your sample needs to be drawn, to whom you should target your questionnaire and how many to issue.

Chapter 5: Techniques for data collection

After deciding on your research approach you will be involved in collecting the data for your research study. If you are collecting 'primary' data (data collected at first hand), you need to undertake certain activities such as inviting your sample to complete the questionnaire, preparing the data summary sheet or taking whatever action is required for your fieldwork. If you are collecting 'secondary' data (data gathered from some other sources), you need to contact those organisations that store the data (if not stored in the library), such as the state and its agencies, statistical offices such as Her Majesty's Stationery Office (HMSO) and the Health and Safety Executive (HSE). Chapter 5 explains the main features of the postal survey and the interview technique, together with showing the advantages and limitations of both techniques.

Chapter 6: Questionnaire construction

This chapter describes and illustrates methods of questionnaire construction: the content of questions, types of questions, question format and the sequence of questions.

Note to students: After constructing your questionnaire, it is strongly recommended to conduct a trial run on the questionnaire before circulating it to the whole sample. This trial is called a 'pilot study'. The pilot study involves testing the wording of the questions, establishing the length of the questionnaire, avoiding ambiguous questions, and suggestions for analysing the data, as well as testing the technique selected for collecting the data. In large research projects such as MPhil or PhD, the researcher should even try to analyse the results of the pilot study to ensure the reliability of data collected. Chapter 6 gives further details on the pilot study.

Chapter 7: Measurements and probability

This chapter prepares the ground for analysis of your results. It is concerned with the nature of measurement in research. It includes the explanation of the four levels of measurement: nominal, ordinal, interval and ratio. The main point to recognise about measurement is that each level of measurement requires a certain type of analysis that is more appropriate than others. This chapter will also explain the meaning of the term 'probability' and its relevance to the analysis of your results.

Chapter 8: Analysis of the results

Once you have collected all the completed questionnaires and/or gathered the archival data, you will be ready for the next stage: the analysis of the data and determining the direction of the study. This stage involves processing the data, putting answers to categories and generally finding out the pattern of the responses. Some results require statistical analysis, as in the case of a large sample survey, and some results involve finding out the trend of the responses, as in the case of in-depth interviews. Chapter 8 gives details on how to analyse the results both manually and with the use of the SPSS (Statistical Package for the Social Sciences) software.

Chapter 9: Structuring and writing the dissertation

After you have completed the literature review and analysed the data, you will be ready to write up the whole dissertation. Writing your dissertation involves reporting and critically appraising the literature review, analysis of the data, discussion and interpretation of your findings. Bear in mind that the writing-up stage can be overlapped with any of the above activities and may start as early as the literature review stage. Chapter 9 provides details on structuring and writing a typical dissertation project.

Chapter 10: Dissertation supervision and assessment

Once you have decided on the topic of your study and your proposal gets approved, your department should then appoint a personal supervisor for you. It is therefore important to know the role of your supervisor and what can be expected from him/her.

This chapter will discuss the basics of what you should expect from your supervisor. It first explains what the role of the supervisor is and what it is not. Second, it illustrates how you may plan your dissertation and finally how you would expect to be assessed in the end.

Reference

Soanes, C. and Stevenson, A. (2004) *Concise Oxford English Dictionary*. Oxford University Press.

Part I

Preparing the ground and reviewing the literature

2 Selecting a topic and writing the dissertation proposal

The first step of the research process involves selecting a research topic and writing your dissertation proposal. This means that you need to do a great deal of reading and clear thinking to identify the problem and your area of interest. This chapter deals with choosing a topic for research and gives guidance on writing your dissertation proposal. The contents of Chapter 2 are illustrated in Figure 2.1.

Choosing the topic

When embarking upon research as part of an undergraduate or a postgraduate study programme, it is important that you pay particular attention to the choice of subject or topic of the research. The choice of topic usually comes from your interest in and value of a particular subject. This interest and value will eventually be developed into a series of questions that you are keen to find answers to. If you are finding difficulty in choosing a researchable topic, you can consider the following:

1 Consulting the library catalogue and inquiring about theses and dissertations, articles in academic journals, reports, books and the like.
2 Using web searching to find areas of interest.
3 Talking about problems and possible topics with your colleagues and/or with your lecturers who are experts in the field.
4 Arranging an informal interview with professionals in the industry and discussing what you should emphasise and what are the possible practical outcomes.

There are a number of criteria that need to be considered when deciding on your research topic. These are summarised below:

1 *A dissertation topic should be realistic.* You need to identify a problem (supported by published materials), investigate the causes and possible solution. You might wish to investigate a problem on site, for example the causes of variation orders and its effect on the project outcome, or the problem of material management on site. Alternatively, the research subject might cover an

Figure 2.1   *Contents of Chapter 2.*

office procedure or the appraisal of a particular system. Here you will be investigating what should be done and what is actually done.

2   *Your topic should be specific and narrow.* For example, if you are conducting a detailed case study, do not investigate all the factors that may influence site productivity as a topic, but rather limit yourself to the influence of financial incentives on productivity. You might be tempted to study job satisfaction in the building industry, but this again is too broad. A better way is to narrow it down and investigate job satisfaction of operatives who are working for small-size firms. Narrowing down the topic can be diagrammed as in Figure 2.2. Bouma and Atkinson (1995, p. 30) comment:

the first thing to do if we are to narrow and clarify a problem question is to 'unpack' it. Most of the starting-points contain many issues and suggest many different avenues of research. The questions we begin with are usually quite complex. They may sound simple, but they are probably far from it. If we are to narrow and focus the issues for research, we have to list the issues involved in the question. We are then in a position to choose from that list, a question that will focus our attention on a narrowed problem.

3   *Your topic should show individuality, that is your personal contribution to the study.* What is new about your investigation? This can take the form of case

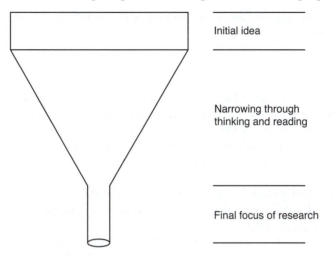

Initial idea

Narrowing through
thinking and reading

Final focus of research

Figure 2.2   *A diagram showing the narrowing down of the research topic.*

studies, a series of interviews, postal questionnaires or analysing archival
data (Chapters 4 and 5 discuss these approaches in detail).
4 *Accessibility of information.* Your topic should be in an area for which you
   can have access to the data necessary for the successful completion of the
   dissertation.
5 *Personal ability.* The subject and extent of the research should be within your
   intellectual and physical resource ability.
6 *Personal interest.* Last but not least, you should be interested in the subject
   of research. It is of no use if you do not like or enjoy the research subject.

The dissertation proposal

After you decide on a topic for research, your dissertation proposal should contain
the following:

1 Working title
2 Purpose (rationale for the study)
3 Research goals
     Aim
     Objectives
     Key questions
     Hypothesis (if applicable)
4 Initial literature review
5 Outline methodology
6 Proposed contents
7 Initial references
8 Work plan

The extent and degree of detail for your proposal should ideally take the following into account.

Working title

A working title is a short line that gives your research a 'direction' and the title might change slightly at the final stages of research. The title should give your research an identity/name that reflects the focal point and area of the research. It should therefore be clear and to the point. There are a number of questions to be borne in mind when selecting a final title. These are:

1 Does the title identify precisely what is being studied?
2 Is the title clear and concise and at the same time sufficiently descriptive to allow for rapid categorisation?
3 Has the title been stripped of superfluous words and redundancy? Phrases such as 'A contribution to . . .' or 'Towards a theory of . . .' are nothing more than padding.
4 Are the key nouns correctly chosen and in the proper order?

(See examples of working titles in Appendix 1.)

Purpose of the research (or rationale for the study)

This should be a one-page discussion of approximately 500–1000 words that sets out (with supporting empirical facts that are fully referenced) the problem and the reason for the proposed study, highlighting the issues to be investigated (see Appendix 1 for examples).

The research goals

This section contains four parts, namely the aim, objectives, hypotheses or assumptions, and key questions.

Aim

Ideally a *one*-sentence aim should be provided, highlighting your ultimate goal. Appendix 1 provides examples of aims but here are some more specimens:

Example 1:   To *provide professional guidelines* to engineers who are required to undertake the role of the project manager.
Example 2:   To *develop a conceptual model* for analysing productivity barriers of subcontracting.
Example 3:   To *develop a theoretical model* for identifying the different factors that may influence the behaviour and effectiveness of project managers.
Example 4:   To *construct a comparative table* showing the difference in

performance between various types of procurement methods.

Example 5: To *design a management system* for improving the safety performance to small-size contractors.

Example 6: To *develop a chart* that demonstrates the strength of the relationship between implementing lean construction initiatives and productivity level on site.

Example 7: To *develop a mathematical formula* to predict the productivity level of various construction techniques.

Example 8: To *construct a scoring matrix* showing the level of performance between management and traditional form of contracts.

Note to students: Notice that the above aims are phrased as if the researcher is seeking to deliver some kind of a 'product' that would benefit the industry and other future researchers, such as to provide professional guidelines, to develop a conceptual framework, to construct a comparative table, to design a management system, to develop a chart, to develop a mathematical formula or to construct a scoring matrix.

In the conclusion chapter, you need to deliver the product that you have aimed for at the start of your research. Appendix 7 shows an example of an achieved aim.

Objectives

Ideally between three and five single-sentence objectives should be developed. Objectives are the breakdown of your aim (sub-aims), which focuses on finding out or establishing certain issues while achieving your aim (see Appendix 1 for examples). The objectives will then pose a number of questions that will form your research questionnaire later in the research process. As shown, try to phrase each objective in the form of:

To investigate . . .
To analyse . . .
To assess . . .
To examine . . .
To compare . . .
To test . . .
To critically appraise . . .
To find out . . .
To evaluate . . .

etc.

Hypothesis

If your research is designed to test or validate a hypothesis or a conceptual theory, or to explain a phenomenon, then a one-sentence main hypothesis needs to be established that should clearly and specifically state the position for the argument or investigation. This main hypothesis can be broken down into a number of sub-hypotheses (see Proposal 2 in Appendix 1).

A hypothesis is a tentative proposition that is a subject of verification through your investigation. Your conclusion will either support or reject your proposed hypothesis, or support part and reject others. Hypotheses can often be formulated as 'if . . . then' statements, or as a hunch that you have about the existence of a relationship between issues or variables. Your hypothesis should also be sharp and specific. Appendix 1 provides various types of hypotheses.

Key questions

A number of 'key questions' need to be formulated in your proposal that would state the position for the argument or investigation. Appendix 1 provides various types of key questions.

Initial literature review

In this part of your proposal you need to expand on the rationale section and write an initial literature review of approximately 1000 words. (See examples of writing-up styles in Chapters 3 and 9.)

Outline methodology and research road map

In this part of the proposal you should highlight your proposed methodology for obtaining the information necessary for the study. Research methods can take many forms (see Chapter 4). At the proposal stage, however, all you need to provide is an outline methodology, for example which academic journals you will concentrate your reading on. If you intend to interview personnel, who will they be and approximately how many of them will you interview?, and so on (see Appendix 1 for examples).

It is strongly recommended to include a road map for your research methodology (see a typical example of a research road map in Figure 2.3 and also Figure 9.2).

Proposed structure of the dissertation

Naturally, you would not be expected to provide the precise structure of your dissertation at this stage, but an initial indication is necessary. So in this part you need to provide the proposed titles of your chapters, which will be subject to verification and can be tweaked at the end. For example:

Chapter 1: Introduction and background to the problem
Chapter 2: Previous project management models
Chapter 3: Apparent advantage and disadvantages of project management
Chapter 4: Research design and methodology

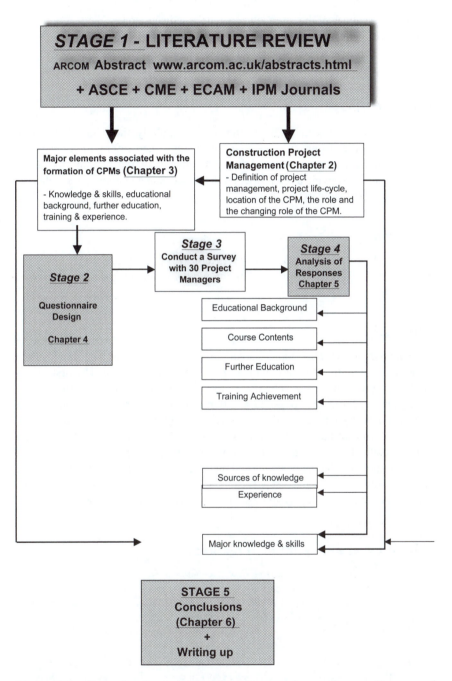

Figure 2.3 *Example of a typical methodology road map. Source: Naoum and Al-Dhyaf (2006).*

Chapter 5: Analysis of the interviews, results and discussion
Chapter 6: Conclusions and recommendations

(See Appendix 1 for more examples.)

Initial references

Details of the core sources of references, particularly those that have been consulted in order to provide the basis of evidence and information necessary to enable the dissertation proposal to be developed, should be indicated. Each reference should provide author, title, publisher, edition and publication data (see Appendix 1 for examples).

Work plan

This should be a simple work plan or timetable. A bar chart of activities over the weeks of study is often helpful, indicating what you intend to do and when (see Figure 10.1).

Summary

Selecting your dissertation topic is an important task. Therefore, you should allow a reasonable amount of time in which to develop your proposal. The first step is to identify areas that have potential and seem interesting to you. Consult your library and read articles, books, dissertations, etc. that are related to your area of interest. Discuss your ideas with your colleagues and/or lecturers. The second step is to write your initial proposal following the instructions given in this chapter (see Appendix 1 for examples). The three most important parts of your proposal are the purpose of study, objectives and methodology. Finally, discuss your initial proposal with your appointed supervisor and make amendments, if required. Start your investigation as soon as you can and stick with your work plan.

References and additional reading

Bell, J. (2005) *Doing Your Research Project: A Guide for First-Time Researchers in Education and Social Science.* Fourth edition. McGraw-Hill International.

Bouma, G. and Atkinson, G. (1995) *A Handbook of Social Science Research: A Comprehensive and Practical Guide for Students.* Oxford University Press.

Howard, K. and Sharp, J. (1993) *The Management of a Student Research Project.* Gower.

Naoum, S. and Al-Dhyaf, S. (2006) 'Formation of Construction Project Managers', CIB W65 conference on building and construction, 10–14 October, Rome, Italy.

Naoum, S., Guowel, G., and Pearson, S. (2011) *Dissertation Guide: Instructions for Preparation, Control and Presentation of the Dissertation.* Department of Property, Surveying and Construction, London South Bank University.

3 Reviewing the literature

The literature review is an essential stage in conducting a research project and amounts, on average, to between 20 and 25 per cent of a dissertation content, although certain dissertation subjects may require a literature review amounting to up to 50 per cent of the content. The literature review involves reading and appraising what other people have written about your subject area. It can be both descriptive and analytical. It is descriptive in that it describes the work of previous writers and it is analytical in that it critically analyses the contribution of others with a view to identifying similarities and contradictions made by previous writers.

There are five main activities involved in undertaking a literature review:

1 knowing the sources of information;
2 understanding how the library works;
3 collecting existing knowledge on the subject, reading and note-taking;
4 systematically organising the literature;
5 appraising and writing up the literature review.

This chapter focuses on discussing the above five activities. The contents of Chapter 3 are illustrated in Figure 3.1.

Rationale for undertaking a literature review

In order to be able to make an original contribution to knowledge in your research area, the literature review should demonstrate that you have a comprehensive grasp of existing knowledge. The literature review serves two purposes. First, it seeks systematic reading of previously published and unpublished information relating to your area of investigation. The gathered information will develop issues and themes and should drive you to the next important stage, namely research design. Second, the literature review will help you to improve your research study by looking into previous research design or questionnaires, which will give you some insights into how you can design your own study more effectively. The authors of past dissertations, theses and published journal articles gave their research work a great deal of thought, and you can frequently benefit from their thinking when

Figure 3.1   *Contents of Chapter 3.*

conducting your literature search. In other words, a literature review attempts to integrate what others have done and said, to criticise previous scholarly works, to build bridges between related topic areas and/or to identify the central issues in a field. The following sections describe the activities involved in undertaking the literature review.

Knowing the sources of information

Starting the literature review process involves the identification of appropriate literature. Generally speaking, there are three types of literature sources available for you to look at. These are primary sources, secondary sources and reference guides.

Note to students: It is strongly recommended that you visit the following link from the ARCOM (Association of Researchers in Construction Management) web site: http://www.arcom.ac.uk/abstracts.html.

This web site address states the following:

> One of ARCOM's most important publications is the CM Abstracts and Indexes. This contains the full titles, authors, abstracts and keywords of articles from several leading Construction Management journals, from recent ARCOM Conference Proceedings, and from PhD theses. The journals currently covered in the database are:

- Architectural Engineering and Design Management
- ARCOM Annual Conferences (since 1997)
- Building Research and Information
- Construction Innovation: Information, Process, Management
- Construction Papers (ceased in 1983)
- Construction Management and Economics
- Engineering, Construction and Architectural Management
- International Journal for Construction Marketing
- International Journal of Construction Education and Research
- International Journal of Disaster Resilience in the Built Environment
- International Journal of Law in the Built Environment
- Journal of Construction Procurement
- Journal of Construction Research (ceased in 2006)
- Journal of Corporate Real Estate
- Journal of Engineering, Design and Technology
- Journal of Financial Management in Property and Construction
- Lean Construction Journal
- Unpublished PhD Theses

Primary literature sources

Primary literature is the most accurate source of information as it publishes original research. The following publications fall within these primary sources.

Academic research journals (refereed)

Refereed journals related to construction publish original research work and technical papers, which usually report innovative developments in the built environment field such as architecture, town planning, engineering, construction and management. By publishing papers from both industry and academia, refereed journals provide an excellent source for discussing recent developments in your field. Listed below are of some of the international refereed journals related to the built environment:

- American Society of Civil Engineers (ASCE), New York:
  - *Journal of Construction Engineering and Management*
  - *Journal of Computing in Civil Engineering*
  - *Journal of Professional Issues in Engineering*
  - *Journal of Environmental Engineering*
  - *Journal of Management of Engineering*
- *International Journal of Urban and Regional Research*
- *Construction Management and Economics*, Reading University
- *Engineering, Construction and Architectural Management*, Loughborough University
- *International Project Management*, Henley College
- *International Journal of Procurement*, University of Glamorgan
- *International Journal of Construction Maintenance and Repair* (now *Construction Repair*)
- *International Journal of Construction Technology*
- *International Construction Law Review*
- *Financial Management of Property and Construction*
- *Economic Journal*

Refereed conferences

The term 'conference' also applies to symposiums and congresses. In many fields, conference proceedings can be a main source of information and the main aim of these conferences is similar to that of academic journals (i.e. discussing current developments in your field of study). Papers published in proceedings contain a collection of themes such as mega projects, developing countries projects, productivity, design, procurement, economics, law, technology, sociology, psychology, organisation, management and many more. The majority of international conference papers are based on 'primary' research and are accepted for publication after they have been refereed by at least two members of the paper review committee. Therefore, the quality of some conference papers can be as good as refereed journal articles. The British Library Lending Division publishes an 'Index' of conference proceedings. Below is a list of some international conference proceedings related to the construction industry:

- Organisation and Management of Construction Symposium (known as CIB W65)
- Procurement Systems Symposium (CIB W92)
- Building Economics and Construction Management (CIB W90)
- Economic Management of Innovation
- Congress on Computing in Civil Engineering (organised by the ASCE)
- The Design and Environment Conference
- International Conference on Computers in Urban Planning and Management
- Association of Researchers in Construction Management (ARCOM)
- Information Technology in Civil and Structural Engineering Design
- International Congress on Construction
- Automation and Robotics in Construction
- International Cost Engineering Council Symposium
- Financial Management of Property and Construction

Dissertations/theses

It is most important for undergraduate, postgraduate and higher degree students to look at other people's dissertations or theses, where appropriate. Dissertations and theses serve two purposes. First, they enable you to have an idea about the content of the work, the standard expected, the methodology adopted and the structure and style of writing-up. Second, you can benefit from the list of references and bibliography that are attached at the back of the work.

Most libraries have an on-site dissertation and thesis collection as well as a borrowing service through inter-library loans. Students registered for higher degrees can obtain a list of theses from the British Library Lending Division (BLLD). Another option for finding out about other theses is to contact academic institutions requesting a list of accepted dissertations or theses. The contact is usually made through the departmental secretary or the academic thesis supervisor. Once you have identified what you want, your library should do the rest by borrowing the material through the inter-library loan service. A dissertation or a thesis may take 4–6 weeks to arrive and overseas PhD theses may take longer.

Reports/occasional papers

Technical reports and occasional papers can be of great use to you because they are comprehensive and often publish up-to-date information. Moreover, occasional papers and reports of certain research groups are sufficiently prestigious for the researchers concerned to favour them as a method of disseminating their results (Howard and Sharp, 1993). Reports and occasional papers fall within a special category and the following institutions publish these sources of information:

- Chartered Institute of Building (CIOB)
- Royal Institute of Chartered Surveyors (RICS)
- Royal Institute of British Architects (RIBA)

- Building Research Establishment (BRE)
- Construction Industry Research and Information Association (CIRIA)

Government publications

Government publications are one of the largest and most important sources of information, especially for those students analysing secondary data. Government documents may be classified as (a) government administration records and (b) research records for specialists, including a considerable number of statistics and data of value to science and business.

Finding your way around government publications can sometimes be complicated and confusing. This is because of the sheer volume of information published under the category of government documents and because they are often placed outside the normal subject index system. For instance, most people ask for government documents by their popular name and not by their official name (the Latham Report instead of *Constructing the Team*, or the Egan Report instead of *Rethinking Construction*, or the Tavistock Report instead of *Communication in the Construction Industry*, and so on). Therefore, the best way to get around this problem is to ask for the monthly list or catalogue of yearly government publications of the UK, USA or elsewhere. For example, in the UK you should be asking for the monthly lists of materials published by the HMSO or the catalogue of British Official Publications not published by the HMSO (Howard and Sharp, 1993).

Secondary literature sources

Secondary literature sources are those that cite from primary sources such as textbooks and newspaper articles.

Textbooks

Most research is initially based on information from books which the researcher has either come across at the proposal stage or found in a dissertation/thesis bibliography. Textbooks are much easier to trace and obtain than other references. However, one significant difference between books and journals is that research work published in a journal is more recent. It takes less time to have a paper published in a journal than it takes to publish a book. A second difference is that journals contain a range of articles, whereas books often deal with a particular issue. In the initial reading phase involving books, more can be gained from reading edited collections as they are likely to contain a wide range of perspectives on a particular subject.

Trade journals, newspapers and magazines

These are mass media sources of information which often summarise research or provide views on a particular subject. It is very useful to refer to these sources at the start of your dissertation. Students often become interested in a particular topic as a result of reading an article in a newspaper, magazine or trade journal. Below are some mass media sources that are related to the built environment:

- *Contract Journals*
- *Building Magazine*
- *Architects Journal*
- *Construction News*

However, caution should be taken in reporting the findings of mass media sources. Such sources are usually non-refereed and may easily distort or exaggerate scientific claims. Remember that most refereed journals' editorial boards practise peer review for the purpose of ensuring high-quality reporting.

Reference guides

Reference guides are very useful sources of information for short and quick answers to basic questions. The function of the reference guides is to introduce the basic information about a particular subject area. Sources that fall within these guides are dictionaries, glossaries, encyclopaedias and handbooks.

Dictionaries and glossaries

These provide a definition of terms and can be useful in helping you clarify your thoughts. Some of the preferred dictionaries are:

- *The Concise Oxford Dictionary*
- *Webster's Third New International Dictionary of English Language*
- *The Random House Dictionary of English Language*

Other specialised dictionaries are *Kister's Dictionary Buying Guide*, the *Penguin Dictionary of Sociology* and *Dictionary of Social Behaviour and Social Research Method*

Encyclopaedias

These give a concise description of the main aspects of a topic. The most up-to-date and authoritative English encyclopaedia is the *New Encyclopaedia Britannica*. Because encyclopaedias can go out of date fairly quickly, most scientific disciplines encourage and support a variety of specialised handbooks.

Handbooks

The function of handbooks is similar to that of encyclopaedias, except that they are more current. Handbooks, however, have limitations in that they are written by and for other scholars with similar interests and vocabularies (Smith, 1991, p. 46). These usually assume that the user understands the methods and logic of particular disciplines, and they may not have subject indexes.

Understanding how the library works

Having identified the sources of information, the next step that you need to take is to know how to find the material. It is absolutely vital that you understand the library and how to use its sources most effectively. Bell (2005, p. 39) lists three important points that you need to bear in mind while conducting a literature research:

1 Find the most relevant published materials quickly.
2 Avoid getting 'bogged down'.
3 Get into the habit of recording information derived from your reading so that it can be easily found and understood weeks, months or years later.

Therefore, you may have to spend a few days getting to know the services offered by your library, what materials it holds and where, as well as the coding or shelving system it uses (usually the Dewey decimal system). Each library should contain the following:

- Library catalogue
- Abstracts/indexes
- Citation indexes
- Microfiche/microfilm
- CD-ROM, on-line database, Internet/World Wide Web, Telnet, JANET/NISS

Library catalogue

This lists all the material which the library has in stock including books journal titles, videos, and so on. Around the late 1980s, most academic libraries had replaced card catalogues with computer-based catalogues. However, they both register the same details. Typical computer-screen information displays record the location of book, title of book, author's name, number of pages, year of publication and library code number. Magazines, journals and newspapers are catalogued in the same way as the books but include detailed information about which issues/volumes the library holds. Issues/volumes of journals that are not held in the library have to have a special reference to inform the user of the closest library which holds that particular journal volume.

Indexes and abstracts

Indexes and abstracts can help you to trace articles in journals. They both give the title, author and issue/volume details, but abstracts also include a short summary, often fewer than 200 words, of the article. An abstract gives you information about the problem and the survey findings. Indexes and abstracts provide not only a short-cut means of access to information, since they curtail endless random searching through periodical titles on the shelves, but also a large number of references which would not be found by such a haphazard method (Haywood and Wragg, 1982). Most abstracting services classify articles in accordance with the subject they cover. The natural way to start your search on a particular subject is, first, to look at the journal abstract/index. Second, study the abstract and find out whether the article is likely to be worth reading or is merely duplicating material already studied. Third, if it is worth reading, you then start searching the volume you need in order to locate the pages of the article in that volume.

Citation index

Citation indexing reports alphabetical lists by author of papers cited in published articles. This source of indexing provides standard bibliographic information on individual articles written in a particular time period. Their permuted subject index classifies each of these articles by significant words used in each article's title, and the citation index lists by author or by referenced articles.

Citation indexing is important because it graphically depicts scientific networks by quantifying who cites whom (Smith, 1991). Almost all scientific articles or reports published at any time and cited during a particular year will have an accompanying bibliographic list of authors, books, articles, reports and the like which cite the article or author. The researcher may then create a snowball sample of citations in a particular area by looking up each new list of citations. For example, if you know that Professor X is an expert on leadership, you could look up his/her name in the Social Science Citation Index to start tracing a collegial network of experts.

Microfiche and microfilm

Most libraries have these facilities, which means that copies of some newspapers, journals and theses are kept on film, either flat (microfiche) or more usually on reels (microfilm). This means that they take up very little room and a great deal of information can be kept in a small space. Moreover, you can read and print out the information on special readers.

CD-ROM

This is 'compact disk read-only memory'. CD-ROMs are like music CDs, but contain other information. They are very important for tracing information for projects. Here, you can put in the subject you are looking for and obtain a list of relevant references. They give the information needed to trace an article, that is the journal you will find it in, the date it appeared, the author and title details. However, some also give the full text of the article, for example *The Times* and *Guardian* newspapers.

Note-taking

It is important to take notes of your literature as it is the best means to recapitulate what you have reviewed. When taking notes, you should focus on the main issues addressed and the main arguments put forward. Dunleavy (1988) comments that, in conducting a literature review, one needs to get away from focusing too single-mindedly on what the authors are trying to say, and instead focus on what one is trying to get out of a source.

In this context, note-taking forms the basis for the construction of a literature review framework and provides the best way of maximising the extraction of information in the initial reading stage. Note-taking provides you with a focused framework and ensures that unnecessary detail is not incorporated into the review. To enable you to get the most out of the literature, it might be useful if you address each piece of literature with the following questions (Kumar, 1995):

1   What do I know already?
2   What am I looking for in this source; what do I think I need?
3   What is useful or different in this source, given my existing knowledge and interest?

It is also useful to consider a form for taking summary notes since its aim is to enable you to put these notes together in a meaningful way. It is common to find students having no difficulty in note-taking but facing considerable difficulty when it comes to putting these notes together to form a literature review. It can be argued that it is the way the students take the notes that causes the problem. Figure 3.2 is a sample form on which to take notes; ideally it should not be more than one page in length and at the most two pages. Use one form for each piece of literature (Kumar, 1995).

Organising the literature review

Note-taking is highly important in building a good research file. The summary and abstract for each article become important for quickly sifting out the irrelevant from the relevant research. For those that appear relevant, you then proceed to read the entire text. Therefore, it is absolutely essential to start, from day one of your research, to maintain a literature file to store the material that you collect. If it is a 4-month dissertation, one large file will probably be enough to store all the information you gather. However, whether it is a dissertation, a thesis or a research project, the principle of structuring the literature file is the same:

1   Subdivide your file into a number of topical areas. For example, suppose you are investigating the factors that affect operatives' productivity in construction sites. In this case, subdivide your manila file into a number of sections. You may create a section on definition and measurement of the term productivity, another section on previous research that investigated the

---

Reference Details
Author(s):
Year of Publication:
Title of Article or Chapter in Edited Book:
Volume and Issue Number (Journals):
Place of Publication (Books):
Publisher (Books):
Page Numbers (Journal and Edited Book Article):
Source (Classification Number and Library Location):

---

1 Main Issues

---

2 Main Arguments

---

3 Research Methodology (if applicable)

---

4 Main Conclusions

Figure 3.2   *Sample summary note-taking form (Kumar, 1995).*

factors affecting productivity rate, another on previous productivity models and so on.

2 In each of these sections you will include all the literature review that falls under the relevant topic area together with your summary note-taking form (see Figure 3.2). Such file(s) will later help you to:

   (a) Suggest hunches and possible research design to test these hunches.
   (b) Intellectually argue the acceptance or refutation of various authors' arguments.
   (c) Define key concepts and derive into logical relationships between these key concepts.
   (d) Write your literature review chapters. After all, your literature chapters will contain the same topic areas as in your file(s).

3 Create an index sheet at the front of the file. This sheet will provide you with a list of all the articles, book chapters and so on that are included in the file. Each piece of literature needs to have a separate code, which will be the same

code as in the index sheet. The purpose of this exercise is to provide you with a clear view of what you have covered and where.

Writing up your literature review

After you have compiled the sources of information you will be ready to construct your literature chapters and critically appraise the information. A critical appraisal is analytical in nature. It critically examines the contribution of other people's work with the view to identifying the following:

1   similarities in the statements made by previous writers;
2   common issue(s) raised by previous writers;
3   differences or contradiction of statements made by previous writers;
4   criticisms made by previous writers.

The following example might serve as a model to show the style of critically appraising the literature review (Chapter 9, p. 132, for another example). In this example, the material is extracted from Chapter 3 of an MSc dissertation that was submitted by Zoë Elizabeth Mulholland (2010). The title of this dissertation is 'An examination of sustainable construction in the recession'. You may not be familiar with the field of study, but the review puts you in the picture as to what is expected from you. Zoë's goal was to investigate whether the drivers and barriers to sustainable construction changed during the recession at the time of writing.

Example of writing a literature chapter: extract from an MSc dissertation by Zoë Elizabeth Mulholland (2010) at London South Bank University

---

Chapter 3 – Literature review into the drivers and barriers to sustainable construction

3.1 Scope of chapter

This chapter critically appraises the literature review, identifying the similarity of statements; common themes; differences and contradictions and criticisms of the body of evidence. It is divided into five main sections, these are: 1) definition of sustainability; 2) background to sustainable construction; 3) evaluating the literature on the drivers and barriers to sustainable construction; 4) the effect of the recession on the construction industry; and finally, 5) critical appraisal of chapter.

3.2 Definition of sustainability

The subject of sustainability has generated a vast amount of literature over the past two decades. As the construction industry contributes to such a large proportion of what is unsustainable in the UK it too has instigated a large volume of research in this area.

The definition of sustainability and sustainable construction has been widely discussed by Waddell (2008), BERR (2009), Lutzkendorf and Lorenz (2005) and Lapinski (2006). Parkin (2000) stated that there are over 200 definitions for 'sustainable development'. The most widely accepted definition is from the Bruntland report (1987) which describes sustainable development as, "development that meets the needs of the present without compromising the ability of future generations to meet their own". It is also widely agreed that sustainability has a triple bottom line: economic, social and environmental (Newport *et al.* 2003). It is only when demands in all three of these areas are met that sustainable development is achieved (See Figure [B]3.1 below). There is much debate about the priority of these aspects or whether they should be treated equal in all instances (Parkin 2000, Newport *et al* 2003, Lutzkendorf and Lorenz 2005, Fergusson, et al 2006, Williams and Dair 2007).

Figure B *The triple circle of sustainablility. Source: Newport, Chesnes and Linder (2003).*

3.3 Background to sustainable construction

Following the Earth Summit held at Rio de Janeiro in 1992, the British Construction Industry Council set a number of goals for the industry, including a 50% reduction in waste on site. The case for sustainable development has been due to the great environmental impact of buildings. In the UK buildings are responsible for almost half of the country's carbon emissions, half the water consumption, one third of waste to landfill and a quarter of all raw materials used in the economy (BERR 2009). As an example, the views of the Royal Institute of Chartered Surveyors on sustainable construction were presented in a tabulated format that illustrated the breadth of issues covered under this heading and the implications of sustainability throughout the construction life cycle. The table highlights the three pillars of sustainability, breaking down each of the stages into their social, economic and environmental impact.

3.4 Drivers and barriers to sustainable construction

3.4.1 Similarities of statements by previous writers

All the major sources in the academic literature agree on the general principles of sustainability, and the majority quote the Bruntland report's definition of sustainable development established in 1987. Similarly nearly all refer to the triple bottom line of sustainability stating an awareness that it relates not only to environmental aspects but also to social and economic viability as well.

Introductions to each paper outline the case for sustainability and its urgency in tackling climate change. The academic literature is also in agreement that the UK is leading the way with ambitious targets for the reduction of CO_2 emissions. The role of the construction industry is widely agreed to be a crucial part in the reduction of CO_2 emissions and each paper identifies a multitude of areas which can be changed from design, construction and operations.

3.4.2 Common issues

Many common drivers and barriers are identified in the literature. Legislation is repeatedly noted as one of the top drivers, which includes local government and planning authorities' conditions for new construction projects. Many sources admit that without such strict measures much of the industry would not be so active in this area. It is thought by some that sustainable construction has reached the stage where it is no longer optional due to the continuing increase in regulations. On the other hand, it is also is highlighted that unless Building Control Inspectors enforce the regulations stringently many non-compliant projects will slip through undetected (Revell and Blackburn 2007).

Company image was also deemed to a major driver in the adoption of sustainable construction (CRiBRE 2009; RICS 2009). Generally three motivations for this were found: organisations' Corporate Social Responsibility policy, sustainability as a marketing tool or the result of peer pressure. However there was disagreement as to whether this resulted in real applications of sustainable construction or more an effort to look green without necessarily making a tangible difference to their carbon emissions or benefits to social well being.

The literature states many, well documented sources for the tangible benefits of sustainable construction. The non-contentious examples are areas such as energy efficiency which can be identified easily within a company's expenses (Financial Executive 2009). However disagreement arises between sources when these benefits are extended to less material benefits such as increased productivity of employees from better designed buildings.

Nearly all articles contend that sustainable construction increases capital costs. The extent of this increase is widely debated and many state this will rapidly decrease over time, with new technology and more efficient solutions. These costs can be mitigated by getting the brief right early in the design and focusing on solutions which have a viable payback period (Richardson and Lynes 2007). A significant outlay in sustainable construction is blamed on renewable energy technologies which are widely reported to be very expensive with extremely long pay back periods. It is also agreed that the additional capital outlay associated with sustainable development is not reflected in the property's value. It is often reported as a significant barrier to the widespread adoption of sustainable buildings and there is no evidence in the literature to suggest that valuations are starting to account for sustainability (Lutzkendorf and Lorenz 2005).

3.4.3 Differences or contradictions of statements by previous writers

Whether customer demand is a driver or barrier was one of the most debated areas. Some schools of thought proclaim there is real demand for sustainable buildings and major clients are driving the green agenda. However there is a similarly strong counter argument that many clients are talking about sustainability but aren't implementing it on their projects. It appears that there is great variation across the industry's clients and there have been changes very recently in customer demand.

3.4.5 Criticisms

The focus of the academic literature is often on the large scale, new build projects where lessons learnt can not necessarily be transferred to the average client's construction experience. One article investigated the barriers and drivers to sustainable construction (Revell and Blackburn 2007) but it focussed on larger firms. All were in agreement that sustainable refurbishment was the industry's greatest challenge. However, much of the research and sustainable construction solutions focuses on new build projects. The issue of improving the existing building stock in the UK receives much less attention.

3.5 The effect of the recession on the construction industry

The construction industry was stated as being very sensitive to the economic climate, often being the worst affected in terms of job losses, decreased activity and duration of downturn (British Council of Offices 2010). Journals and trade publications lamented the cyclical nature of construction activity resulting in the continual boom to bust effect. It was agreed, due to the complex interactions between the various environmental forces acting on construction, the impact of each recession was different. It was widely agreed that the current recession was deep, global and affecting all sectors across the construction industry.

Conflicting views arose in the literature as to how construction was affected in the recession, in terms of training, innovation and adopting new practices. Some sources stated that the recession caused cost cutting of projects, reductions of scope and quality with many of the skilled professionals being lost through redundancies. The other school of thought was that in fact the industry could benefit from leaner times, forcing the industry to be more efficient with its resources and more innovative with its solutions (Hillebrandt 1995).

Recent evidence

The sources available for recent evidence were very restricted but a consensus was starting to form: the pace of sustainable construction may be slowing but it was not being abandoned. Several articles suggested that the volume of construction had reduced but that which was continuing was not necessarily any worse in terms of quality or sustainability. In contrast some state that sustainability was still on the agenda despite the economic downturn but it was questionable whether these statements of commitment would actually translate into action.

Conflict in opinion was revealed when the RICS Economics survey (2009) stated that 90% of its respondents said that the relevance of sustainability had not changed or had in fact increased in importance. In contrast, the recent Building Saint-Gobain (2009) online survey reported that 58% felt it had decreased significantly in light of the recession. Another disagreement in the recent evidence was the willingness of the market to pay a premium for sustainable construction. Again the Building Saint-Gobain (2009) survey reported negative responses with 85% stating affordability of sustainable construction as a major barrier. But the JLL survey (2008) recorded 65% of their respondents in the property sector were willing to pay more for a sustainable building.

All evidence points towards sustainable construction continuing to grow in importance not only to Government but to clients across all sectors. It was agreed that the UK Government would continue strengthening regulations irrespective of the recession. Even where there was scepticism to current projects including high standards of sustainability there was unanimous agreement that in five years time it would be of much greater importance. Essentially construction is seen in the literature as being only at the beginning of the curve towards adopting sustainable construction.

3.6 Critical appraisal of chapter 3

In this final section of the chapter, Zoe inserted a critical appraisal section (approximately 500 words) to discuss the implications of the information provided in that particular chapter on her investigation.

3.7 References

BERR (2009), http://www.berr.gov.uk/whatwedo/sectors/construction/sustainability/page13691.html. Accessed 1 February 2009.

Blackburn, R. (2007), The business case for sustainability? An examination of small firms in the UK's construction and restaurant sectors, *Business Strategy and the Environment,* Vol. 16, pp.404–420.

British Council for Offices (2010), *The Role of Property in Recessionary Cycles.* www.bco.org.uk/research/researchreports Accessed 27 March 2010.

Bruntland Commission (1987), *Our Common Future.* Oxford: Oxford University Press.

Building (2009) http://t35ts1t32010.uat.building.co.uk/news/short-term-fears-voiced-over-sustainability-in-the-recession/3135025.article. Accessed 20 April 2010

CRIBE (2009), *Greening the commercial property sector: a guide for developing and implementing best practice through the UK leasing process.* http://www.cf.ac.uk/archi/cribe.php. Accessed 28 March 2010.

Fergusson, H. and Langford, D.A. (2006), Strategies for managing environmental issues in construction organizations, *Engineering, Construction and Architectural Management,* Vol.13 (2), pp.171–185.

Financial Executive (2009), Recession-proof your building, *Financial executive,* May 2009. www.Financialexecutive.org

Hillebrant, P.M. (1995), *The Construction Industry In and Out of Recession.* London: Macmillan Press.

JLL (2008), *Perspectives on sustainability,* October 2008. www.joneslanglasalle.com. Accessed January 31 2009.

Lapinski, A. (2006), Lean processes for sustainable project delivery, *Journal of Construction Engineering and Management,* October 2006

Lutzkendorf, T. And Lorenz, D. (2005), Sustainable property investment: valuing sustainable buildings through property performance assessment, *Building Research & Information,* Vol. 33 (3), pp.212–234.

Parkin, P. (2000), Sustainable development: the concept and practical challenge, in Proceedings of the Institute of Civil Engineers, *Civil Engineer,* Vol.138, p.3–8.

Revell, A. and Blackburn, R. (2007), The business case for sustainability? An examination of small firms in the UK's construction and restaurant sectors, *Business Strategy and the Environment,* Vol. 16, pp. 404–420.

Richardson, G.R.A. and Lynes, J.K. (2007), Institutional motivations and barriers to the construction of green buildings on campus, *International Journal of Sustainability in Higher Education,* Vol. 8 (3), pp. 339–354.

RICS (2008), Q1 Global Property Sustainability Survey, *RICS Economics.* www.rics.org/economics. Accessed 31 January 2010.

Newport, D., Chesnes, T. and Lindner, A. (2003) The "environment sustainability" problem: ensuring that sustainability stands on three legs, *International Journal of Sustainability in Higher Education,* Vol. 4 (4), pp. 357–363.

Waddell, H. (2008), Sustainable construction and UK legislation and policy, in Proceedings of the Institute of Civil Engineers, *Civil Engineering,* Vol. 162, pp. 53–62.

Williams, K. and Dair, C. (2007), What is stopping sustainable building in England? Barriers experienced by stakeholders in delivering sustainable developments, *Sustainable Development,* Vol. 15, p. 135–147.

Note to students: The above example attempts to demonstrate 12 fundamental aspects of a good literature review:

1 A clear literature title.
2 Division of chapters into sections: it starts with 'Scope of chapter' and ends with 'Critical appraisal'. (See Chapter 9, p. 135, for another example.)
3 Sifting of information. This means that the student included materials which are directly related to her study.
4 Clarity in writing: it is precise and clear in presenting other people's work.

5   Clearly appraising the common issues raised by previous writers in the field, as well as the similarities and differences among them.
6   Coherence in writing: the material is presented in an orderly, logical progression to facilitate understanding and good reading.
7   Good grammar and punctuation.
8   Where relevant, the use of accurate linking phrases such as 'in contrast', 'it has been reported by', 'according to', 'there is much debate about', 'another school of thought suggests', 'all evidence points towards', 'conflict in opinion was revealed when', 'two sources, namely . . . and . . . admitted that' and so on.
9   The inclusion of a diagram, such as the one shown in Figure B3.1 to clarify the point to be made as well as to make the reading more interesting. You may also wish to include other interesting exhibits and illustrations such as tables, charts, conceptual frameworks and so on that were developed by previous writers.
10 Acknowledging the work of others. Good citation and accurate referencing. Naturally, this list of references would be part of the overall referencing list, which would be inserted at the end of the dissertation. However, some students may prefer to include the reference list at the end of each chapter.
11 A good balance of old and new references.
12 A good balance of sources. For example, it includes material published by:
    – refereed journals;
    – conference proceedings;
    – reports;
    – secondary sources such as textbooks,
    – web sites.

Note to students: For more insight into Zoe's research, please read the publication by Naoum and colleagues (2011).

Summary

The literature review is one of the earliest stages in the research process and it amounts to a significant proportion of a dissertation content. This review basically searches for material that is relevant to the subject of your dissertation with the intention to describe and analyse what has been written by others. It can take some time to get to grips with. Hence, it is advisable to allow sufficient time to cover the activities involved in undertaking a literature review. These activities are (a) knowing the sources of information, (b) understanding how the library works, (c) note-taking, (d) organising the literature review and (e) appraising and writing up the literature review.

References and additional reading

Bell, J. (2005) *Doing Your Research Project: A Guide for First-Time Researchers in Education and Social Science*. Fourth edition. McGraw-Hill International.

Cooper, H. (1998) *Integrated Research: A Guide for Literature Reviews*. Second edition. Sage.

Dunleavy, P. (1988) *Studying for a Degree in the Humanities and Social Sciences*. Macmillan.

Haywood, P. and Wragg, E. (1982) *Evaluating the Literature*. Rediguide 2, School of Education, University of Nottingham.

Howard, K. and Sharp, J. (1993) *The Management of a Student Research Project*. Gower.

Kumar, S. (1995) Undertaking Literature Review. Unpublished paper. London South Bank University.

Mulholland, Z.E. (2010) 'An examination of sustainable construction in the recession', MSc dissertation, Department of the Built Environment, London South Bank University.

Naoum, S., Mulholland, Z., Fong, D. (2011) 'Sustainable Construction in the Recession'. 11th World Sustainable Building Conference SB11, October, Helsinki, Finland. Paper ID 1666853.

Smith, H.W. (1991) *Strategies of Social Research*. Holt, Rinehart and Winston.

Part II

Research design and methodology

4 *Approaches to data collection*

Once you have determined the purpose of your study and have completed a thorough literature search, you should be ready to design your research in detail. Research design is an action plan for getting from 'here' to 'there', where 'here' may be defined as the initial set of questions to be answered, and 'there' is some sort of conclusion (answers) about these questions. Between 'here' and 'there' may be found a number of major steps, including the collection and analysis of relevant data (Yin, 1994).

This chapter will review the various approaches to data collection. It first explains the difference between 'quantitative' and 'qualitative' research. Second, it explains the two main approaches to data collection known as 'fieldwork' and 'desk study', and will discuss the survey approach, the case study approach, action research and archival data collection. The contents of Chapter 4 are illustrated in Figure 4.1.

Research strategy

One of the problems of reading about research methods and techniques is the terminology. Writers use terms that may be incomprehensible to other people. In order to avoid confusion, it may be helpful to define the various terms as I go along. Here, research strategy can be defined as the way in which the research objectives can be questioned. There are two types of research strategies, namely 'quantitative research' and 'qualitative research'. Deciding on which type of research to follow depends on the purpose of the study and the type and availability of the information that is required.

Quantitative research

Quantitative research is 'objective' in nature. It is defined as an inquiry into a social or human problem, based on testing a hypothesis or a theory composed of variables, measured with numbers and analysed with statistical procedures, in order to determine whether the hypothesis or the theory holds true (Creswell, 1994). Quantitative data are, therefore, not abstract; they are hard and reliable; they are measurements of tangible, countable, sensate features of the world (Bouma and Atkinson, 1995).

Figure 4.1   *Contents of Chapter 4.*

Quantitative research is selected under the following circumstances:

- when you want to find facts about a concept, a question or an attribute;
- when you want to collect factual evidence and study the relationship between these facts in order to test a particular theory or hypothesis (see Proposal 2 in Appendix 1).

Chapters 6 and 7 provide examples of questionnaire construction as well as types of measurement. But here are some quantitative questions:

- What were the programmed and the actual construction duration of the project (in weeks)?
- What was the final cost/sq. m. of the project?
- What method of construction did you use to build the project?
- How many fatal accidents has your company been involved with over the past 3 years?

Note to students: The techniques and tools that are commonly used in data collection are described in Chapter 5.

Placement of the theory in quantitative research

In quantitative study, the hypotheses, research questions and objectives can be better understood when they are grounded in a theoretical framework. The concept of a theoretical framework is explained in detail in a later section. However, at this point, I would like to discuss the term 'theory'. A theory is commonly understood to have certain characteristics. Kerlinger (1979), cited by Creswell (1994, p. 73), defined a theory as:

> a set of interrelated constructs (variables or questions), that presents a systematic view of phenomena by specifying relationships among variables, with the purpose of explaining natural phenomena. Here, the systematic view might be an argument, a discussion, or a rationale that helps explain (or predict) phenomena that occur in the world.

A theory can be introduced as:

*   *A series of hypotheses/sub-hypotheses in the form of 'if . . . then' logic statements*. For example, a proposition that the more money you offer to operatives, the more productive they become is a theory.
*   *A hunch*. For example, a hunch about the quickest method (method A or method B) to build a building of type X is a theory.

In quantitative studies one uses a theory deductively and places it towards the beginning of the plan for a study: the objective is to test or verify a theory, rather than develop it. One thus begins the study advancing a theory, collects data to test it, and reflects on whether the theory was confirmed or unconfirmed by the results in the study. The theory becomes a framework for the entire study, an organising model for the research questions or hypotheses and for the data collection procedure (Creswell, 1994). (Proposal 2 in Appendix 1 is an example of theoretically based research.)

Qualitative research

Qualitative research is 'subjective' in nature. It emphasises meanings, experiences (often verbally described), description and so on. The information gathered in qualitative research can be classified under two categories of research, namely exploratory and attitudinal.

Exploratory research

Exploratory research is used when you have a limited amount of knowledge about your topic. Here, the interview technique is usually selected as a method of data collection (see Chapter 5). The purpose of exploratory research is intertwined with the need for a clear and precise statement of the recognised problem. Researchers conduct exploratory research for three interrelated purposes: diagnosing a situation, screening alternatives and discovering new ideas (Zikmund, 1997). For instance, personnel research managers often conduct exploratory research as a diagnostic tool to point out issues of employees' concern or to generate possible explanation for motivational patterns. For example, preliminary interviews with employees may be utilised to learn current 'hot' issues, as well as concerns about bread-and-butter issues such as wages, working conditions and career opportunities.

The raw data provided in exploratory research will be exactly what people have said (in interview or recorded conversation) or a description of what has been observed.

Questionnaire construction is discussed in Chapter 6, but the following discussion summarises the format of questions that can be asked in the exploratory study. Creswell (1994, p. 72) writes: 'One typically finds research questions (not hypotheses) written in exploratory research. These research questions assume two levels: (1) one or two "grand tour" questions followed by (2) no more than five to seven "sub-questions".' On the assumption that the researcher will comply with these two levels, the following ideas for a qualitative study may prove helpful:

- Begin the research questions with the word 'What' or 'How'. Tell the reader that the study will do one of the following: discover, explain or seek to understand, explore a process, describe the experiences.
- Pose questions that use non-directional wording. These questions describe, rather than relate variables or compare groups. Delete words that suggest or infer a 'quantitative' study, words with a directional orientation, such as 'affect', 'influence', 'impact', 'determine', 'cause' and 'relate'.
- Expect the research questions to evolve and change during the study, a thought also consistent with the assumption of an emerging design. Often in qualitative studies the questions are under continual review and reformulation.
- Use open-ended questions without reference to the literature or theory unless otherwise dictated by a qualitative design type.

The following is an example of exploratory research questions (Goodman and Adler, 1985, p. 2, cited by Creswell, 1994, p. 72):

Example – Explaining or seeking to understand

How are (these) conceptions of social studies played out – or not played out – in classroom practice? (A grand tour question) . . . How is each setting organised? (The beginning of sub-question) . . . What kind of interpersonal dynamics exist? . . . How do the students, co-operating teachers, faculty members, and pupils act? . . . What activities occur in each setting? What topics are discussed, and what information, opinions, and beliefs are exchanged among the participants?

Attitudinal research

Attitudinal research is used to 'subjectively' evaluate the 'opinion', 'view' or the 'perception' of a person, towards a particular object. The term 'object' is referred to as an 'attribute', a 'variable', a 'factor' or a 'question'. Chapters 6 and 7 provide examples of questionnaire construction as well as types of measurements. But here are some specimens of subjective questions:

- Do you think that 'lack of worker's motivation' is a factor that can significantly affect productivity on site?
- Yes/No/Difficult to say.
- Safety officers should have the power to stop operatives from work if they see them working in an unsafe manner, such as without helmet. Please express your level of agreement.
- 1. Agree strongly 2. Agree 3. Disagree 4. Disagree strongly 5. No opinion.
- Please indicate which of the following factors is most important to motivate operatives to work harder on site, which comes next in importance, which is third and so forth.

Job security	1st rank, 2nd, 3rd, 4th, 5th
Money	1st rank, 2nd, 3rd, 4th, 5th
Work condition	1st rank, 2nd, 3rd, 4th, 5th
Job interest	1st rank, 2nd, 3rd, 4th, 5th
Prosperous job	1st rank, 2nd, 3rd, 4th, 5th

Note to students: The data gathered under the qualitative research can later be 'quantified' to some extent but a qualitative approach tends to value the data as 'qualitative' (Coolican, 1993).

Placement of the theory in qualitative research

In qualitative research the use of theory is less clear than in quantitative design because there is no standard terminology or rules about placement. A theory may be placed at the beginning of the research or emerge during the data collection and analysis phase, or be used relatively late in the research process as a basis for comparison with other theories. However, the placement of theory in qualitative research usually tends to be towards the end of the study. Therefore, the end product of qualitative research will be throwing up hunches and hypotheses which can be tested more rigorously by further quantitative research.

Creswell (1994) identifies some principles to observe about using a theory in the qualitative approach: (a) employ it in a manner consistent with the type of qualitative design, (b) use it inductively so that it becomes not something to test, but rather something to develop and be shaped through the process of research, (c) create a visual model of the theory as it emerges and (d) if used at the end of the study, compare and contrast it with other theories.

Comparing quantitative and qualitative research

From the above discussion you may have noticed a number of contrasting features of quantitative and qualitative research. The difference between quantitative research and qualitative research is rather like the difference between counting the shapes and types of design of a sample of green houses as against living in them and feeling the environment. The difference between each one may be somehow quantifiable but such measurements will not convey the importance and the special impact of some over others.

Bryman (1988) provides a useful list of differences between the two research strategies. Table 4.1 includes some of the important dimensions. Naturally, the focal point of any research is its outcome. Although Table 4.1 shows distinctive features of the two strategies, the relationship between theory/concept and research strategy in terms of verifying the theory or concept, rather than expecting a theory to emerge from the data, is not as clear-cut as is sometimes implied.

Approaches to data collection

The approach to be adopted for conducting the research depends on the nature of the investigation and the type of data and information that are required and available. For the student reading this book, there are two approaches to data collection, namely fieldwork (primary data collection) and desk study (secondary data collection), both of which are described below.

Fieldwork research

In this book, the term 'fieldwork research' refers to the methods of primary data collection used by the researcher and must not be confused with the definition of

Table 4.1 *Some differences between quantitative and qualitative research (Bryman, 1998)*

	Quantitative	Qualitative
1 Role	Fact-finding based on evidence or records	Attitude measurement based on opinions, views and perceptions measurement
2 Relationship between researcher and subject	Distant	Close
3 Scope of findings	Nomothetic	Idiographic
4 Relationship between theory/concepts and research	Testing/confirmation	Emergent/development
5 Nature of data	Hard and reliable	Rich and deep

field research as 'the study of people acting in the natural courses of their daily lives'. Here, fieldwork can be associated with three practical approaches:

1 the survey approach;
2 the case study approach;
3 the problem-solving approach (action research).

Note to students: Other approaches, such as observational and experimental studies, are also useful to know, but they are of very limited use to the level of students reading this book. They usually require long periods of time in the 'field' and emphasise detailed evidence.

The survey approach

Surveys are used to gather data from a relatively large number of respondents within a limited time frame. A survey is thus concerned with a generalised result when data are abstracted from a particular sample or population (see Chapter 5, Sampling, p. 57) There are two types of surveys available: the descriptive survey and the analytical survey.

1 The descriptive survey aims to answer such questions as How many? Who? What is happening? Where? and When? It deals with counting the number of respondents with certain opinions/attitudes towards a specific object. The counting can be analysed later to compare or illustrate reality and trends; for example, the number of respondents in the survey that answered 'Yes' to the question, 'Should safety officers have the power to stop operatives from work if they see them working in an unsafe manner?' or the number of contractors that have more than five site accidents each year.
2 The analytical survey aims to establish relationship and association between the attributes/objects of your questionnaire, that is how often an attribute is associated with another attribute within the sample questionnaire. For example, you might find that most of the respondents who answered 'Yes' to the question whether 'workers' motivation affects site productivity' are operatives, and the majority who answered 'No' are site managers. In this sense, you may conclude that site managers are not aware of how important motivation can be to improve site productivity. This relationship is shown in Figure 4.2.

   In the example in Figure 4.2, the category of respondents is known as an 'independent variable' and attitude/views towards motivation is known as a 'dependent variable'. In other words, the attitude of respondents is dependent upon who the respondents are. In some surveys you might find a significant relationship between the independent and dependent variables, and in others you will find no significant relationship (see Chapter 8). The terms 'dependent' and 'independent' variables are described further in the case study approach.

Figure 4.2   *A diagram showing relationship between the independent and dependent variables.*

Note to students: There are situations when you need to explain why a particular phenomenon is taking place. For example, in analysing the results of accidents on site, you may find a drop, over a period of time, in the number of accidents that the contractors have recorded in their books. You may need to explore why this is happening. Is it the contractor's policies with regard to safety which made the record go down, or is it the provision of new health and safety regulations? The answers to these types of questions, although they can be assumed by the researcher and they are acceptable at the level of students reading this book, may not be totally adequate. Therefore, the 'why' questions and the 'cause and effect relationship' can be better explained and interpreted by designing an 'analytical case study'.

The case study approach

Case studies are used when the researcher intends to support his/her argument by an in-depth analysis of a person, a group of persons, an organisation or a particular project. As the nature of the case study focuses on one aspect of a problem, the conclusion drawn will not be generalised but, rather, be related to one particular event. This is not to say that the case study approach is of limited value. On the contrary, it provides an in-depth analysis of a specific problem.

There are three types of case study designs:

1   The descriptive case study, which is similar to the concept of the descriptive survey (i.e. counting), except it is applied on a detailed case(s).
2   The analytical case study, which is similar to the concept of the analytical survey (i.e. counting, association and relationship), except it is applied on a detailed case(s).
3   The explanatory case study, which is the theoretical approach to the problem. It explains causality and tries to show linkages among the objects of the study. It asks why things happen the way they do. It also suggests that a single cause can have a specific effect. In other words, the researcher collects facts and studies the relationship of one set of facts to another, with the hope of finding some causal relationship between them.

Note to students: If the sample is large, then the relationship can be tested statistically. If the sample is small, then the relationship can only be discussed 'intellectually', which is acceptable for the level of students reading this book.

An example of an explanatory case study is when you have a hunch (related to a hypothesis or a theory) that the larger the project is, the more difficult it becomes to control the construction operations and, subsequently, the project will overrun its schedule. This relationship/hypothesis is shown in Figure 4.3.

As mentioned earlier, analytical research means that you have identified an element that causes, affects or has an influence on another element. This is basic to the logic of a hypothesis (Bouma and Atkinson, 1995). The element that does the causing is called an 'independent variable'. The element which is acted upon, produced or caused by the independent variable is called a 'dependent variable'. In Figure 4.3, the size of project is an independent variable and overrun on time is the dependent variable.

However, time overrun is not determined solely by the size of the project. Projects can also overrun because of the selection of an inappropriate procurement method, client variation orders, client inexperience, environmental factors such as weather, and industrial factors such as strikes. Each of these causes will have a greater or lesser effect depending on its strength. Therefore, you need to construct a theoretical or a conceptual framework. Sometimes a model is used instead of, or interchangeably with, a theoretical framework. Using the example above, the model in Figure 4.4 is possible.

In Figure 4.4 the three variables – client experience, project complexity and size of project – are the independent variables and are related to the dependent variable, time overrun. One of the independent variables is seen to be negatively related and the other two are positively related to the dependent variable. Here,

Figure 4.3 *A diagram showing the relationship between an independent variable (size of project) and the dependent variable (overrun on time).*

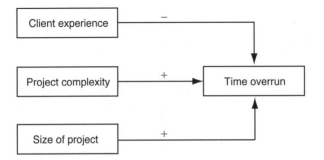

Figure 4.4 *A diagram showing three independent variables and one dependent variable.*

the negative sign means that, the more experienced the client is with the building process, the less chance there is that the project will overrun. Another possible model would be that shown in Figure 4.5.

The variables in Figure 4.5 are related in such a way that client experience, project complexity and size of project affect the selection of procurement method, which in turn affects time overrun. Here, procurement method is working as an intervening variable. An intervening variable is a process that helps to explain linkages between the dependent and independent variables and can cause the relationship between them to change.

Bouma and Atkinson (1995, p. 45) comment that the possibilities of such diagrams/models are endless. They write:

> While the most complex theories can be diagrammed, most research projects deal with only one small aspect of the whole diagram. It is often a useful discipline to diagram more than you plan to study in order to show where the proposed research fits in the larger frame of reference.

The theoretical/conceptual framework can:

- be a self-designed framework which can be formed as a result of a literature search coupled with informal interviews with persons who have a wealth of knowledge about the subject area;
- use a previous theoretical/conceptual framework; or
- modify an existing framework.

Note to students: There are situations, however, in which the 'how' and 'why' questions can be answered by a survey and/or a case study. For example, how and why individuals within the organisation become leading managers can be studied by a survey together with a case study. The survey can examine the leadership pattern of organisations, showing that people with decisive characteristics are more likely to become leaders. In contrast, the case study might examine how particular leaders conduct their public relations to achieve their goal.

Figure 4.5   *A diagram showing three independent variables, one intervening variable and one dependent variable.*

Problem-solving approach (action research)

With the survey and the case study approach, the researcher tends not to affect or interfere with what is being studied. In the problem-solving approach (also named action research), the researcher reviews the current situation, identifies the problem, gets involved in introducing some changes to improve the situation and, possibly, evaluates the effect of his/her changes. This type of research is more attractive to practitioners, industrialists and students from the professional backgrounds who have identified a problem during the course of their work and wish to investigate and propose a change to improve the situation.

Examples of problem-solving research include changing organisation policy towards promotion, designing a new information flow system, recommending a new system for measuring the quality management of the organisation and the like (see Proposal 3 in Appendix 1, as an example).

It has to be stressed that, whatever idea is to be recommended, it must be original and practical. Moreover, the dissertation project must be structured and written as an academic piece of research and not as a project report.

Secondary data collection

The data collected using the above three approaches (surveys, case studies, problem-solving) are called 'primary' data because they are obtained first hand. The data collected using the desk study approach are called 'secondary' data because the data are obtained from other sources. Secondary data can be stored in either a statistical or a descriptive format. Secondary information has some distinctive advantages over primary data collection effort. Stewart and Kamins (1993, p. 37) note:

> The most significant of the advantages of the secondary data are related to time and cost. In general, it is much less expensive to use secondary data than it is to conduct a primary research investigation. This is true even when there are costs associated with obtaining the secondary data. When answers to questions are required quickly, the only practical alternative is to consult secondary sources. If stringent budget and time constraints are imposed on primary research, secondary research may provide higher quality with a new research project. Secondary data also may provide a useful comparative tool. New data may be compared with existing data for purpose of examining differences or trends.

Statistical format

In construction-related research, the word 'statistical' refers to official statistics collected by the state and its agencies. These statistics are available in all public libraries and in most university libraries. The sources that publish this official information include institutions such as:

- British Research Establishment
- Her Majesty's Stationery Office
- Chartered Institute of Building
- Royal Institute of British Architects
- Royal Institute of Chartered Surveyors
- Construction Industry Research and Information Association (CIRIA)
- Building Research Establishment
- Health and Safety Executive (HSE)

Generally speaking, the above institutions assemble the data in two ways, namely through registration or self-survey. As far as the registered information is concerned, all construction-related companies are required to provide information to the government by law. Therefore, the researcher can at any time make use of this data to show 'what is happening'. On the other hand, government bodies conduct their own routine surveys to collect data and publish them at regular intervals, say every year. For example, in the fourth proposal shown in Appendix 1, the student intended to look in depth at the type of accidents within the construction industry and compare them with other industries. He, therefore, brought together empirical evidence related to accidents on site gathered from several sources. For instance, the student used the statistical data provided by the Health and Safety Executive (Statistical Services Unit) in Liverpool to analyse figures and present them in graphs. This method allowed the student to make a critical examination of the data (see Table 8.5 on p. 99 for further details on analysis).

Descriptive documents

The other method for conducting secondary data research is to analyse and critically appraise the contents of an archival document. This is similar to appraising previous literature and can include diaries, newspapers, observations and so on.

Secondary data are usually processed before the researcher starts to make use of them. Therefore, the researcher should take absolute care when using them. Below are some questions that ought to be considered when using secondary data:

- Is the material factually accurate?
- Is the material reliable? Would it have been the same if it had been collected by anyone else?
- Is it systematic, providing a complete account of what it describes? What is lacking?
- Why was it collected?
- Is the material representative?

Of course, there is no way that the researcher can answer any of these questions with certainty, but they should be borne in mind. Nevertheless, most of these questions have to be asked when collecting primary data as well.

After gathering the information that is required for your investigation you will then need to analyse it. Chapter 8 explains various methods of data analysis.

Summary

This chapter reviewed the various approaches to data collection in construction. It first distinguished between quantitative and qualitative research. Quantitative research is an objective measurement of the problem, investigating facts and trying to establish relationships between these facts, whereas qualitative research is a subjective assessment of a situation or problem, and takes the form of an opinion, view, perception or attitude towards objects. An object is referred to as an attribute, variable, factor or question.

This chapter also explained the approaches to data collection that are suitable for the level of students reading this book. It explained the survey approach, the case study approach, action research and archival data collection approach.

References

Bouma, G. and Atkinson, G. (1995) *A Handbook of Social Science Research: A Comprehensive and Practical Guide for Students*. Oxford University Press.

Bryman, A. (1988) *Quantity and Quality in Social Research*. Unwin Hyman.

Coolican, H. (1993) *Research Methods and Statistics in Psychology*. Hodder & Stoughton.

Creswell, J. (1994) *Research Design: Qualitative and Quantitative Approach*. Sage.

Goodman, J. and Adler, S. (1985) Becoming an elementary social studies teacher: A study in perspectives. *Theory and Research in Social Education*, 13(2), 1–20.

Kerlinger, F.N. (1979) *Behavioral Research: A Conceptual Approach*. Holt, Rinehart, and Winston.

Stewart, D. and Kamins, M. (1993) *Secondary Research: Information Sources and Methods*. Second edition. Sage.

Yin, R. (1994) *Case Study Research: Design and Methods*. Sage.

Zikmund, W. (1997) *Business Research Methods*. Dryden Press.

5 Techniques for data collection

After you have decided on the type of data to be collected (quantitative, qualitative or both), and have also decided on the research approach (survey, case study, action research or analysing archival data), you will be in a position to think seriously about the technique for collecting the data. This chapter will explain the main features of two major research techniques available to elicit data and information from respondents. These are the postal questionnaire and the personal interview. It has to be stressed, however, that data collection does not necessarily depend on one method or technique. Some research depends solely on one method of data collection but others do not. In other words, it is possible for you to conduct a postal questionnaire and a case study, or to conduct interviews in addition to a postal questionnaire, or whatever. It is also possible that your dissertation questionnaire includes quantitative questions as well as qualitative ones. Your decision will depend on your judgement as to which method or techniques will best obtain the information you need in order to achieve the purpose of your study. Whatever decision you make, you need to consult your supervisor before going ahead with it. The contents of Chapter 5 are illustrated in Figure 5.1.

Postal questionnaire

The postal questionnaire is probably the most widely used data collection technique for conducting surveys. It is most suited to surveys whose purpose is clear enough to be explained in a few paragraphs of print, in which the scheme of questions is not overelaborated. Postal questionnaires have been widely used for descriptive and analytical surveys in order to find out facts, opinions and views on what is happening, who, where, how many or how much. Almost all postal questionnaires have 'closed-ended' questions that require a specific response such as 'yes' or 'no' or ranking the importance of factors (see Chapter 6 for details).

The main advantages of postal questionnaires are:

- *Economy.* Postal questionnaires are perceived as offering relatively high validity of results because of their wide geographic coverage. As a result, they are more suited to assembling a mass of information at a minimum expense in terms of finance, human and other resources.

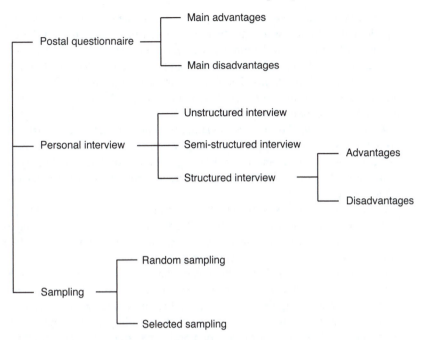

Figure 5.1   *Contents of Chapter 5.*

* *Speed.* Postal questionnaires are certainly a quick method of conducting a survey. If administered properly, the bulk of the returns will probably be received within 2 weeks. However, time must be allowed for late returns and responses to follow-up attempts. For example, if there is a lack of response to the first return of replies (beginning about 2 weeks after initial posting), a reminder needs to be sent to those who have not yet returned the questionnaire. Therefore, a period of about 4 weeks needs to be allowed in your programme of work from the date of the initial mailing to the commencement of the final analysis.

* *Consultation.* In certain cases respondents may not have the information to hand, particularly when the questions are of a quantitative nature, and the respondent may need to consult a document or a colleague in order to give accurate answers. Examples are questions such as 'When was the project built and what was its building cost?' or 'How many fatal accidents has your organisation been involved in over the past 5 years?' Such questions may have to be answered in the respondent's own time, rather than provided on the spot as is usually associated with interviews. However, such a problem can be overcome in the interview if the questionnaire is posted to the respondent in advance of the interview.

The main limitations of postal questionnaires are:

- *Must contain simple questions.* The postal questionnaire is suitable only for simple and straightforward questions which can be answered with the aid of easy instructions and definitions. The questions should be very carefully worded and free from faults such as ambiguity, vagueness, technical expressions and difficult questions. These faults can affect the results of the postal questionnaire even more seriously than when conducting an interview (see the following section, 'Personal interview').
- *Inflexible technique.* Postal questionnaires are inflexible in the sense that they do not allow the opportunity for probing. In other words, the answers have to be accepted as final and there is no opportunity to clarify ambiguity or to appraise the non-verbal behaviour of respondents, though the latter can sometimes create bias.
- *Accuracy.* Respondents may answer generally when you are seeking a response on a specific level of analysis. People may also answer according to what they think you want to hear. They may answer according to their public profile rather than the underlying corporate reality.
- *No control over respondents.* This means that, although you state in your questionnaire that a particular person should complete the questionnaire (such as the marketing director, managing director or site agent), there is no guarantee that this statement will ensure that the right person completes the questionnaire. However, this is less of a problem than not getting a response at all, given the fact that response rates for postal surveys usually range between 40 and 60 per cent.
- *Industry fatigue.* Companies receive a steady stream of questionnaires and the pressures of modern business mean that, for many organisations and individuals, students' questionnaires have a lower priority.

Note to students: Some of the limitations of the postal questionnaire can be overcome by supplementing it with personal interviews.

Personal interview

The personal interview is another major technique for collecting factual information as well as opinions. It is a face-to-face interpersonal role situation in which an interviewer asks respondents questions designed to elicit answers pertinent to the research hypothesis. The questions, their wording and their sequence define the structure of the interview (Nachmias and Nachmias, 1996). The interview technique is suitable under the following circumstances:

- When the people being interviewed are homogeneous and share the same characteristics.
- When you know enough about your interviewee so you ask only what is important and know how to ask it.
- When interpersonal contact is essential to explain and describe the questions.
- When a case study needs to be investigated in detail asking questions such as how and why things had happened the way they did.

- When the research requires an explanation of why the respondents are answering or feeling the way they do, that is more than a Yes or No, or Agree or Disagree answer.

Interviews can take three forms: unstructured, structured and semi-structured. Some research may require one form of interview, although others may require a combination of the three forms. There are many other terms in use to distinguish between what are called here structured and unstructured interviews. For example, there are formal and informal, inflexible and flexible, standardised and unstandardised, controlled and uncontrolled interviews.

Unstructured interview

This form of interview uses 'open-ended' or 'open' questions and the questionnaire is often pitched at a very general level so that the researcher can see in what direction the interviewee takes things in their response. It is usually conducted with qualitative research (see 'Qualitative research' in Chapter 4).

Unstructured interviews can also be conducted at the beginning of any research (also known as exploratory interviews) when the researcher knows little about his/her subject area. However, in this type of interview you need to have a clear research outline that you are familiar enough with to carry the general points around in your head. Here, there is no set order or wording of questions, no schedule and you are not looking for the same information from each person. It is purely an exploratory exercise. For example, suppose you are studying the factors that affect job satisfaction for construction operatives and you wish to explore your thinking around this research outline through informal interviews. On your first interview, the operative may focus his/her discussion around salary, job security and promotion as motivating factors affecting his/her satisfaction with the job. On your informal interview with the second, third or fourth operatives, you will seek to find out whether the same factors apply to them as well, and if there are other factors that need to be added. For instance, other operatives may add leadership, working environment and the organisation itself. At the end of the unstructured interviews you will probably end up with a list of 10 factors which you will then examine on a wider sample through structured interviews or a postal questionnaire.

Note to students: Some students rely solely on two or three exploratory unstructured interviews. This is not enough from which to draw firm conclusions.

Semi-structured interview

This is more formal than the unstructured interview in that there are a number of specific topics around which to build the interview. This form of interview uses 'open' and 'closed-ended' questioning but the questions are not asked in a specific order and no schedule is used. Your task is to discover as much as possible about the specific issues related to your subject area. Merton and Kendal (1946) state four distinguished characteristics of the semi-structured interview or, as they named it, a focused interview:

1   It takes place with respondents known to have been involved in a particular experience.
2   It refers to situations that have been analysed prior to the interview.
3   It proceeds on the basis of an interview guide specifying topics related to the research hypotheses.
4   It is focused on the respondents' experiences regarding the situations under study.

Semi-structured interviews start by asking indirect questions in order to build up a rapport with the respondent and then explore the specific issues that the interviewer has in mind. Suppose you are investigating the factors which cause conflict between managers and the site agents. You may start by asking the site agents 'What sort of problems do site agents have in getting along with their managers?' and 'What sort of disagreement do you have with your site manager?' You can then move on to ask more formalised questions such as 'Have you ever had any disagreement with your manager over the following: (a) allocation of resources, (b) scheduling, (c) overtime pay, (d) promotion?'

In the semi-structured interview, the interviewer has a great deal of freedom to probe various areas and to raise specific queries during the course of the interview. For example, the first question above can be probed by asking 'In what way do site managers try to restrict your work?' or 'Do any of your colleagues have the same problem?'

Structured interview

In the structured interview, questions are presented in the same order and with the same wording to all interviewees. The interviewer will have full control on the questionnaire throughout the entire process of the interview. In this technique the questioning may start with some 'open' questions, but will soon move towards a 'closed' question format. Nachmias and Nachmias (1996, p. 20) cited three assumptions of the structured interview:

1   That for any research objective, the respondents have a sufficiently common vocabulary so that it is possible to formulate questions which have the same meaning for each of them.
2   That it is possible to phrase all questions in a form that is equally meaningful to each respondent.
3   That if the meaning of each question is to be identical for each respondent, its context must be identical and, since all preceding questions constitute part of the context, the sequence of questions must be identical.

The main advantages of the structured interview therefore are:

- The answers can be more accurate.
- The response rate is relatively high (approximately 60–70 per cent), especially if interviewees are contacted directly.
- The answers can be explored with finding out 'Why' the particular answers are given.

Note to students: There is another data collection technique, which is known as the 'telephone interview'. The rules and techniques that are applied to telephone interview are similar to face-to-face interviews. It incurs high cost but it is a quicker way to find a respondent to interview. It may not be as detailed as face-to-face interviewing; however, technological changes and improvements in communication equipment have made telephone interviewing easier, especially when researchers use random-digit dialling and computer-assisted telephone interviewing (see Nachmias and Nachmias, 1996).

Sampling

Once you have decided on the technique for collecting your fieldwork data and have thought about what you want to ask, you should be ready to decide on the characteristics of the respondents. In all cases a sample has to be drawn from its population. The term 'sample' means a specimen or part of a whole (population) which is drawn to show what the rest is like. For instance, if you are conducting a postal survey then you need to obtain a list of respondents which is known to fall into the category of your survey (survey sample). If you are conducting case studies interviews then a relatively small number of cases (interview sample) is used for inferences to all cases (a population).

Selecting the research sample is very important and great care must be taken when choosing the type of sample design. The researcher has to ensure that the characteristics of the sample are the same as its population and act as representative of the population as a whole. Usually, drawing a representative sample is done either randomly or non-randomly. The term 'random' means selecting subjects (respondents) arbitrarily and without purpose.

Designing the research sample can take many forms, each of which is suitable to a particular situation. Listed below are some of the types of sampling designs available to the researcher:

- non-random accidental sampling;
- non-random purposive sampling;
- simple random sampling;
- systematic random sampling;
- stratified random sampling.

Detailed description of the above types of sampling design is beyond the scope of this book. Students conducting an MPhil or PhD research should know about these types and ought to consider reading the appropriate parts of the references on sampling procedures provided on page 61. However, for the purpose of this book, you need to know that there are two types of sampling: random sampling and selected sampling.

Random sampling

This type of sampling can be used when specifics about the characteristics of the sample are not essential, such as background of respondents, size of company and type of work. However, there are two main criteria that you need to take into consideration when selecting your sample. First, what do you want to know? Second, about whom do you want to know it? Both of these questions can be answered by referring back to the purpose of your study, that is your aim, objectives and hypothesis (or key questions).

In order to draw a random sample you need to follow two steps:

1 Identify the population from which the sample is to be drawn. This means obtaining a list of names and addresses of, say, top contractors operating in the Greater London area. Such names and addresses can be obtained from your direct personal contacts or from organisations and references such as the Building Federation, Chartered Institute of Building and Royal Institute of British Architects.
2 If the list is small, you may be able to send your questionnaire to all the names identified in your list. If the list is long, you then need to devise a method of random selection which ensures that each subject (in this case contractor) has the same probability (chance) of selection. In other words, adopt a random numbering technique to select a sample. For example, if you have a list of 400 contractors and you want a sample of 80, you might select every fifth name on the list.

Selected sampling

This type of sampling is usually chosen with the interview approach. It begins by choosing a list of names and addresses of participants with specific characteristics, for example the top contractors who are offering alternative procurement methods and undertaking refurbishment work for commercial clients. All other contractors will be excluded from the survey. Consider the study by Naoum and Langford (1987) entitled 'Management contracting: the client views'. A structured interview questionnaire was used to obtain the clients' view of management contracting and to compare the management contracting system with the traditional form of contract, having in mind clients' needs in terms of function, cost, speed and aesthetics. This section is not intended to be a thorough treatment of questionnaire construction and administration, as this is covered in Chapter 6. However, it is important to show the questionnaire that Naoum used when interviewing the clients in order to follow the discussion. Table 5.1 provides some of the questions asked. The following procedure was used by Naoum when selecting the 10 clients:

Table 5.1 *Question to clients on management contracting (MC) versus traditional contracting*

Questions	Yes	Same	No
Is MC more risky to clients?			
Is MC more profitable to the contractor?			
Does MC involve fewer claims?			
Is MC more flexible to variations?			
Does MC allow an earlier start on site?			
Is MC quicker during construction?			
Is MC more reliable in predicting the build time?			
Is MC cheaper?			
Is MC more reliable in estimating the building cost?			
Does MC provide more control over subcontractors?			
Does MC exercise more control over construction tasks?			
Does MC provide a better building design?			

1 The name of clients and their addresses were identified from the management contractors who were interviewed in phase one of the research.
2 Names of persons who were suitable to participate in the research were identified through telephone conversations with the client organisations.
3 The 10 clients selected for the interviews were homogeneous and shared similar characteristics. They were all large organisations, were very experienced with the building process and, most importantly, all undertook different types of work under different contractual arrangements. There were, however, differences in that some clients were private organisations and others were public agencies. Moreover, given the nature of their business, some clients had complex organisational structures whereas others had simple ones.
4 A structured interview questionnaire was designed and posted prior to the interview.
5 The interviews provided some freedom to probe certain areas and raised specific queries during the course of the interview. More specifically, 'Why do you feel that way?' and 'Why do you hold that view?' or 'How did this happen?'

In this study, a selected sample of clients was thought to be more appropriate than a random sample because of the nature of the study. If the interviews are based on people who are very different in characteristics, philosophy and experience, the questions will have different meanings for each of them. The answers, therefore, may be ambiguous for the subject under investigation. However, this does not mean that you are not permitted to have a sample of different characteristics. Your research design may require you to compare the views of two groups of people who have different backgrounds; for example, comparing the views of quantity surveyors and clients on the concept of value management technique.

Summary

This chapter discussed the main features of the postal survey and the personal interview together with showing the advantages and disadvantages of both techniques (see Table 5.2 for summary). The postal questionnaire is an impersonal

Table 5.2 *Comparison between a postal survey and interview technique*

	Features	Interviews	Postal questionnaire
1	Identity of respondents	Known	Unknown
2	Interaction between interviewer and respondent	Close	Distant
3	Time involving the researcher	Long time to go through the interview	Short time
4	Cost	High	Significantly lower than the interviews
5	Sample	Small	Large
6	Quality of information	Deep and detailed	Rich
7	Skill and experience	The interviewer needs to have the skill to ask questions and, if necessary, to probe	No skill required
8	Control of the process	High	Low
9	Flexibility	Allows great flexibility to reword questions and clarify terms that are not clear	Rigid. The answers are accepted as they are
10	Analysis of the results	Difficult and becomes complicated in the unstructured interviews	Easy to analyse
11	Interviewer bias	The flexibility of interviews allows for bias. Sometimes the non-verbal communication or behaviour of the interviewee may mislead the interviewer to incorrect judgement	If sample is selected appropriately, there should be no bias

survey technique that is most suitable for a descriptive or analytical survey. Its main advantages are cost-effectiveness, speed of process and that respondents can consult others for information. Its main limitations are that it must contain simple questions, it is inflexible and it gives no control over respondents.

The personal interview is a face-to-face situation that is most suitable for case study research and studies that require respondents with homogeneous characteristics. Interviews can take three forms: unstructured, semi-structured and structured. The main advantages of personal interview are knowing the identity of respondents, interaction between interviewer and respondent, that it allows probing, that the quality of information is deep and detailed, and that the interviewer has a high level of control over the interview process. The main limitations of the personal interview are high cost, long process time, that the sample can be small and difficulty in analysing the information.

References and additional reading

Barnett, V. (1991) *Sample Survey Principles and Methods*. Arnold.

Bouma, G. and Atkinson, G. (1995) *A Handbook of Social Science Research: A Comprehensive and Practical Guide for Students*. Oxford University Press.

Jolliffe, F. (1986) *Survey Design and Analysis*. Ellis Horwood.

Merton, R. and Kendal, P. (1946) The focused interview. *American Journal of Sociology*, 51, 541–557.

Moser, C. and Kalton, G. (1985) *Survey Methods in Social Investigation*. Gower.

Nachmias, C. and Nachmias, D. (1996) *Research Methods in the Social Sciences*. Fifth edition. Arnold.

Naoum, S. and Langford, D. (1987) Management contracting: The client views. *American Society of Civil Engineers. Journal of Construction Division*, September.

Stewart, D. and Michael, K. (1993) *Secondary Research: Information Sources and Methods*. Second edition. Sage.

6 Questionnaire construction

Chapter 5 introduced several techniques for gathering information. As discussed, the selection of the technique depends largely on your choice of the research approach. For instance, if your research requires you to conduct case studies, then the interview technique is more appropriate than the postal questionnaire, and if your study seeks to survey the opinion of top contractors operating in London, then the postal questionnaire will be more appropriate and feasible than interviews. After deciding on the technique, your next step is to construct your questionnaire.

The foundation of all questionnaires, whether to be mailed or to be used for interviewing, is the questions. At first, the order and wording of the questions are not crucial. Your aim is to list the ideas which can be developed into a questionnaire at a later stage. The principles that you need to follow in constructing your questionnaire are shown in Figure 6.1.

Figure 6.1 shows that, during the research process, the research objectives are translated into specific questions. Therefore, while thinking what item or question to include in your questionnaire, you should ask yourself the following:

- Which objective is the question related to?
- Is the question relevant to the aim of the study?
- Is the question relevant to the research hypothesis?
- Can the answer be obtained from other sources?

This chapter describes the stages for questionnaire construction and administration. It describes and illustrates (through examples) the types of questions, question format and typical questionnaires. It also provides criteria for writing the questions. The contents of Chapter 6 are illustrated in Figure 6.2.

Note to students: A typical questionnaire format can be seen in Appendix 2.

How to construct a questionnaire

There are three fundamental stages that you should take in constructing your questionnaire:

Figure 6.1 *A diagram showing that during the research process, research objectives are translated into specific questions.*

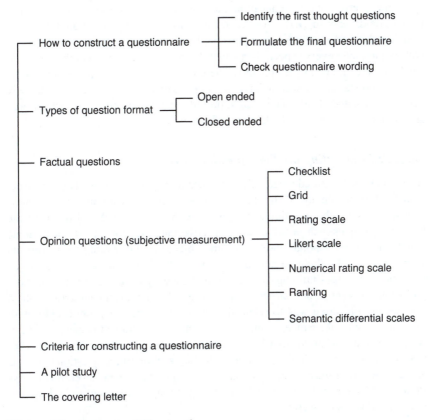

Figure 6.2 *Contents of Chapter 6.*

1   identifying the first thought questions;
2   formulating the final questionnaire; and
3   wording of questions.

Stage 1: identifying the first thought questions

Before constructing your questionnaire, you should go back to your proposal and the literature file and start formulating the 'first thought' list of questions. At this stage, the order and wording of the questions are not crucial. Your aim is to write down all possible questions (say, 20–30 questions) which are related to your research (you will edit and order them later). Suppose you are investigating whether the characteristics of site managers have an effect on project performance. You will be thinking of asking certain types of questions and not others. Whatever questions you intend to ask, they should not be arbitrary and need to be based on your literature review. For example, you may not include in the first thought questions a question about the site manager's favourite location of work, but you are expected to include a question about his/her educational achievement. The reason for this is either that you are assuming that location of work has nothing to do with time overrun but that educational achievement has, or that previous studies in other fields have supported the second assumption. Moreover, should you ask a question about the site manager's personal life? This may just be relevant. But if you start to cover every aspect, then you will end up with a very lengthy questionnaire which could be rather hopeless. Therefore, it is absolutely important that, at the proposal stage, you need to have the purpose of your study specific, narrowly defined and stated clearly. This should provide you with a more focused research and help you to formulate the final questionnaire more easily.

Stage 2: formulating the final questionnaire

After you have identified the first thought questions, you will be ready to construct your final questionnaire. To do that, you need to introduce a number of sections or categories for the questionnaire (say, four to six sections) and try to fit the first thought questions in these sections. Give these sections a title or a theme which should correspond closely with the objectives. For example, in Proposal 1 (in Appendix 1), there were two objectives. The first objective was to survey large private house-building companies and investigate the company business philosophy, organisational structure, marketing information and marketing policy. The second objective was to relate the companies' marketing philosophy with their financial performance. From these objectives, the student began to think of what to ask and what not to ask. He constructed the questionnaire with six sections to correspond with his objectives. The first section of the questionnaire was named 'General Information'. The second section was named 'Overall Business Philosophy' and here he listed six issues that he thought important and relevant to ask. These six issues were:

1   Type of business
2   Business philosophy
3   Management philosophy on products
4   Marketing plan
5   Management philosophy on the market
6   Management success criteria

These items or ideas were not introduced arbitrarily but were based on his background literature review (see Table 6.1).

Stage 3: wording of questions

After deciding what to ask, you should then check how you have asked them. The last section of this chapter gives details on criteria for constructing the questionnaire, but here is a summary:

- Your questions/questionnaire should be short but comprehensive.
- Avoid leading questions.
- Avoid double questions.
- Avoid presuming questions.
- Avoid hypothetical questions.
- The questions must not be ambiguous.
- The questions should be logical in their sequence.
- The questionnaire must be attractive in appearance.

Note to students: Examining other questionnaires to identify possible clues, through which to construct yours, is essential at this stage. This means that you should look at good questions or questionnaires in books, journals, dissertations, theses and so on and try to copy the ideas. Remember, authors of past work have given their research a great deal of thought, and you can frequently benefit from their thinking when designing your questionnaire. For instance, question 3.2 of section 3 in Appendix 2 is a modification of a similar research project which was conducted in the manufacturing industry. The student fine-tuned the wordings to suit his field of investigation. Provided that you make a reference to other people's work, you will not be penalised.

Types of questions

Questionnaires are classified into two types: the 'open' form or unrestricted type, and the 'closed' form or restricted type. Open questions seek to encourage the respondent to provide free responses. For instance, the question 'What do you personally feel are the most important factors that make workers work harder?' is an open-ended question designed to study people's opinion. Oppenheim (1996, p. 112) notes:

Table 6.1   *Questionnaire related to marketing*

Please respond to the following questions by ticking beside the option (letter) which best fits your company

---

SECTION – OVERALL BUSINESS PHILOSOPHY

1   **What business are you in?**
   (a)   We build houses.
   (b)   We build homes.
   (c)   We market homes.

2   **In the house-building cycle, what action best describes your firm's business philosophy?**
   (a)   We first determine customers' wants; and then design the product types and packages to satisfy those wants.
   (b)   We first start to build the estate; and then work out how best to sell the product.

3   **What is the management's philosophy on products and markets?**
   (a)   Management primarily thinks in terms of selling current and new products to whoever will buy them.
   (b)   Management thinks in terms of serving a wide range of markets and needs with equal effectiveness.
   (c)   Management thinks in terms of serving the needs and wants of well-defined markets chosen for their long-term growth and profit potential for the company.

4   **Does management develop different offerings and marketing plans for different segments of the market?**
   (a)   Yes.
   (b)   Sometimes.
   (c)   No.

5   **Which of the following best describes top management's philosophy guiding the firm's current marketing effort?**
   (a)   Customers will favour those products that are affordable and therefore the main task of management is to pursue improved production.
   (b)   Customers will not buy enough of the organisation's products unless the organisation makes a substantial effort to stimulate their interest in its products.
   (c)   The key of achieving organisational goals consists of the organisation's determining the needs and wants of target markets and adapting itself to delivering the desired satisfactions more effectively than its competitors.

6   **Top management's focus is on _____ (please print a, b or c)**
   (a)   Cost (i.e. how to do things cheaply and well).
   (b)   Sales volume (i.e. maximise sales targets).
   (c)   Profit (i.e. maximise profit).

Open or free-answer types of questions are not followed by any kind of choice, and the answers have to be recorded in full. In the case of a written questionnaire, the amount of space or the number of lines provided for the answer will help to determine the length and fullness of the responses we obtain. Inevitably, some of this richness is lost when the answers are classified later, but it is useful to report a few such answers in the final report to give the reader some of the flavour of the replies. Statistical tabulations are important and must remain our first aim, but they make dull reading.

The main advantages of the open type of questions are therefore:

1 They give the respondent the opportunity to express his/her views. Once the respondent understands the theme of the investigation, he/she can let the thoughts roam freely, unencumbered by a prepared set of replies.
2 They are easy to ask.
3 They are more appropriate to construct with interview questionnaires, but can also be used in postal surveys. During the interview, the interviewer has a great deal of freedom to probe various areas and to raise specific queries during the course of the interview.
4 They are useful to adopt when sensitive information is required from the respondent.

Open questions can, however, present problems. As the open question offers no direct clues and is broad based, predictably this type of questionnaire is more difficult to analyse and interpret. Therefore, some form of content analysis is required for open questions (see Chapter 8).

By contrast, closed questions often require a short response in the form of Yes or No, Agree or Disagree, Important or Not Important, and so on. Closed-ended questions are easy to ask and quick to answer, they require no writing by either respondent or interviewer, and their analysis is straightforward (Nachmias and Nachmias, 1996). Their major drawback, however, is that they may introduce bias, either by forcing the respondent to choose from given alternatives or by offering the respondent alternatives that might not have otherwise come to mind.

The appropriateness of either a closed-ended or open-ended question depends on a number of factors. Paul Lazarsfeld (1944) suggested the following considerations to determine appropriateness of which type of question to ask:

- the objective of the questionnaire;
- the respondent's level of information about the topic in question;
- the extent to which the topic has been thought through by the respondent;
- the ease with which respondents can communicate the content of the answer or the extent to which respondents are motivated to communicate on the topic.

Factual questions

This chapter has so far discussed the type of questions. The rest of the chapter will explain and illustrate the different formats for asking the questions. I will start with the factual questions.

Factual questions are mostly designed to elicit information related to the following:

1   Facts related to the background of an individual or organisation. Most ques-
    tionnaires, whether for descriptive or analytical purposes, almost certainly
    begin by asking factual questions such as:
    (a) What is your position within the organisation?
    (b) How many professional employees work within the organisation?
    (c) Which type of projects is your firm specialised in?
    (d) What is the annual turnover of your organisation?
2   Facts related to events or projects. For instance, the questionnaire in Table 6.2
    contains questions which are designed to find facts about the characteristics
    of projects and their performances. In this example, the researcher's aim
    was to investigate the difference in performance of projects delivered by a
    management contract and the traditional form of contracting. A theoretical
    model was formulated and a number of sub-hypotheses were proposed. In
    order to test the sub-hypotheses, factual data were collected from previously
    completed projects and the performance of these projects was measured
    objectively.

Note to students: It is extremely difficult to determine causality in such studies unless a detailed case study is undertaken or a controlling variable system is used. This means you ought to be selective in your sample. For example, you may need to study certain categories of clients or projects and exclude others. In this way you will be limiting the variables that determine causality. Nevertheless, at the level of students reading this book, if some kind of relationship is established between the variables, then that should be sufficient. For MPhil/PhD level an in-depth investigation to causality is necessary; for example, follow-up interviews should be conducted with those involved in the study to explain how and why certain events took place. Otherwise, causality can be best studied in an experimental type of research such as laboratory and social behaviour research. As mentioned earlier, these are outside the scope of this book. They basically involve validating the hypotheses under real test.

3   Facts gathered from secondary data. As mentioned in Chapter 5, secondary
    data are available in two formats: statistical and descriptive. For example,
    in Proposal 4 shown in Appendix 1, the student examined and analysed the
    type of accidents within the construction industry using material which was
    published by the HSE Statistical Services Unit in Liverpool (see the HSE

Table 6.2 *Project details questionnaire*

SECTION 1 – QUESTIONS RELATED TO PROJECT CHARACTERISTICS

1 What was the project type? (Please tick the appropriate option)
- (a) Housing
- (b) Industrial
- (c) Commercial
- (d) Other type (please specify)

2 What was the type of construction?
- (a) Steel structure frame
- (b) Reinforced concrete
- (c) Both (a) and (b)
- (d) Other (please specify)

3 How was the project funded?
- (a) By private funds
- (b) By public funds
- (c) By both funds
- (d) By other funds (please specify)

4 What was the gross floor area in square metres? (Please state)

5 Was it a new-build project, refurbishment or both? (Please state)

6 How many main subcontractors were involved in the project? (Please state)

SECTION 2 – QUESTIONS RELATED TO THE CONTRACTUAL ARRANGEMENTS

7 What procurement method was selected for the project?
- (a) Traditional
- (b) Management contracting
- (c) Design and build
- (d) Project management
- (e) Other method (please specify)

8 What was the tendering arrangement?
- (a) Negotiation
- (b) Open tendering
- (c) Selective tendering
- (d) Two-stage selective tendering
- (e) Serial or continuous
- (f) Other method (please specify)

9 What was the tendering document?
- (a) BOQs/drawings
- (b) Drawings/specification
- (c) Approximate BOQs
- (d) Other document (please specify)

SECTION 3 – QUESTIONS RELATED TO PROJECT PERFORMANCE

10   **Please give the overall contractual price tender accepted for the building in £s.**

11   **Please give the actual price on completion of building in £s.**

12   **If the actual cost exceeded the estimated, was it authorised by the client?**
(a) Yes
(b) No

13   **If your answer to question 12 above is Yes, how much of the amount was authorised by the client?**
(a) All of the amount
(b) Some of the amount (please state amount)

14   **Please give the programmed duration of the project (in weeks).**

15   **Please give the actual duration of the project (in weeks).**

16   **If the actual duration exceeded the programmed, was the extension authorised by the client?**
(a) Yes
(b) No

17   **If your answer to question 16 above is Yes, how many weeks were authorised by the client?**
(a) All extension requested
(b) Some of the requested extension (please state)

---

record in Appendix 4 as a typical example). From these statistics, the student compared the accident rate of the construction industry with four other major industries within the UK. He also took the accident statistics for the construction industry and separated them into their elements and components to show their type and relation to employees. Analysis of these factual records was then presented in graphical forms (see Figure 8.2 on p.100).

Opinion questions (subjective measurement)

There are several formats in which opinion type of questions can be asked:

- checklist
- grid
- rating scale
- Likert scale
- numerical rating scale
- ranking
- semantic differential scales

Checklist

This type of question is essentially a list of items, about themselves, an organisation or an event, that respondents are offered to mark or tick. It is a straightforward means of collecting information and the data can be analysed easily. For example, a question may be a list of management techniques and the respondent is asked to tick which of these techniques are used by his/her organisation. It may be a list of motivational factors and respondents are asked to tick which of these apply to them, and so on.

The checklist questions are specially designed for a group of respondents who have accurate information and can answer the questions with a high degree of certainty. For example, a respondent may be asked a question on a specialised area, such as: 'Over the next 5 years or so, do you expect the use of value management to:

1   Increase a lot
2   Increase a little
3   No change
4   Decrease a little
5   Decrease a lot?'

The checklist format is a quick format but can be rather rigid. The response to each item has not a degree of intensity, but a dichotomy. As an attribute, it is either applicable or not. Two examples of checklist questions are illustrated in this chapter. Table 6.1 was an exhibit of a checklist of questions taken from a dissertation topic on marketing related to Proposal 1 in Appendix 1. Table 6.3 is another exhibit in which a checklist is used to find out the level of knowledge people have on a particular subject.

Table 6.3   *Which of the following problems do you think need to be overcome in relation to the project management system?*

Please tick one or more of the following

No universally accepted definition of project management.	☐
No standard form of project management.	☐
Defining responsibilities on members of the project management team.	☐
Controlling the work packages of the project.	☐
Associated problem of communication.	☐
Higher cost associated with the project management system.	☐
Attitude of personnel involved in the project management project.	☐
Others (please state).	☐

Table 6.4   *Below are some well-known procurement methods that can be used to deliver projects according to client criteria. Please tick those procurement methods that you think are best to achieve each criteria listed*

	Procurement method		
Criterion	Traditional	Construction management	Design and build
Speed of total process Building complexity Building quality Cost of change Degree of price certainty Functionality Buildability			

Grid

A grid is an elaboration of the checklist format, except it provides answers to two or more questions at the same time (see example in Table 6.4).

Rating scale

The rating scale is one of the most common formats for questioning respondents on their views or opinions of an object, event or attribute. Like the grid, rating scales can be regarded as an elaboration of the checklist format, except the respondent has the choice to express his/her degree of agreement or disagreement on a particular scale. The response categories of such questions are called quantifiers: they reflect the intensity of the particular judgement involved. The following are some common sets of response categories:

1 Strongly agree (5 points)	1 Of great importance	1 More	1 Too little
2 Agree (4 points)	2 Of some importance	2 Same	2 About right
3 Neither/nor (3 points)	3 Of no importance	3 Less	3 Too much
4 Disagree (2 points)	4 Do not know		
5 Strongly disagree (1 point)			

1 Very satisfied	1 Very favourable	1 Very bad
2 Fairly satisfied	2 Favourable	2 Bad
3 Fairly dissatisfied	3 Not favourable	3 Would not matter
4 Very dissatisfied		4 Fairly good
5 Very good		
6 It would depend		

The numerical number shown beside the first category represents the intensity of the response. These are not usually shown in the questionnaire but are included here for your own use at the analysis stage.

Table 6.5 shows an extract from a questionnaire which was designed to investigate the views of the industry on factors affecting productivity on construction

Table 6.5 *Below are a number of factors which can have an impact on site productivity. From your experience, please express your opinion on how important each factor can be on influencing productivity. (Please tick the appropriate box)*

Factors influencing site productivity	Of great importance	Of some importance	Of no importance
1 Head office factors			
Delegation of responsibilities			
Integration of project information			
Project planning			
Scheduling of project activities			
Level of authority			
Supervision of subordinates			
Communication between head office and site			
Involvement of site managers in contract meetings			
Characteristics/attitude of site personnel			
The decision-making process			
2 Resource management effectiveness			
Procurement of materials			
Site programme			
Accuracy of the technical information			
Appropriateness of tools to be used for the tasks			
Knowledge of project technology			
Management interference on workmanship			
Site layout			
3 Motivational factors			
Promotion of employee			
Resentment regarding company policy			
Incentive schemes for good performance			
Opportunities to exercise skill/knowledge			
Management response to settle employee's grievances			
Workers uncertainty about career prospects			
Work environment			
4 Education and training			
Experience of employees			
Contract administration skill			
Knowledge of scientific techniques			
Training on new technology			
Availability of multi-skilled project personnel			

sites. Respondents were asked to rate various factors they considered important. This type of rating is also called 'matrix rating'.

With the rating scales, it is your task to decide the number of scale points to use. Moser and Kalton (1993, p. 359) write:

> If the scale is divided too finely the respondents will be unable to place themselves within the scale, and if too coarsely the scale will not differentiate adequately between them. Often five to seven categories are employed, but sometimes the number is greater. The choice between an odd or even number depends on whether or not respondents are to be forced to decide the direction of their attitude; with an odd number there is a middle category representing a neutral position, but with an even number there is no middle category, so that respondents are forced to decide to which side of neutral they belong. Another factor to take into account in fixing the number of categories is that respondents generally avoid the two extreme positions, thus effectively reducing the number they choose between.

Likert scale

This type of scaling is similar to the rating scale, except the questions consist of attitudinal statements on the survey object (say attitude to job satisfaction) ranging from one extreme of favourableness to the other. Table 6.6 is an exhibit of a Likert scale questionnaire extracted from Mullins's (2010) book, *Management and Organizational Behaviour*.

Numerical rating scale

The numerical rating is another common questionnaire format. In this format, respondents are asked to give scores on an analogy, a service or an event. The rating may be out of 100, out of 10, out of 5 and so on. Examination marking is a typical example of a numerical rating scale. Table 6.7 is an exhibit of a subjective way to tell the respondent's opinion on the criteria that are used in assessing project performance.

Ranking

The ranking format is used when the respondent is asked to place a set of attitudes or objects in ranking order indicating their importance, priorities or preferences. For example, in a survey on the level of job satisfaction, respondents were asked to rank various dimensions they considered important about being in their jobs (see Table 6.8). There are, however, particular limitations to the number of rankings most people can be expected to carry out. Under normal survey conditions, to put 10 objects in rank order is probably as much as can be asked (Oppenheim, 1996). Therefore, for a large number of objects you need to ask the respondents to rank for you a number of factors (say five factors) out of many factors as in the example shown in Table 6.9 on p. 79.

Semantic differential scales

Diagrammatic rating scales is another means of measuring intensity of judgement and the semantic differential is the most popular form of this type of scaling. The technique was developed by Osgood (1956) to investigate the perceived meaning of various concepts. In this method, the respondent is asked to indicate his/her position on a seven-point bipolar scale defined with contrasting adjectives at each end. It can best be applied when the perceptions of different groups on a particular matter need to be compared. Examples could be good/bad, strong/weak, satisfied/dissatisfied.

The seven-point bipolar scale can be presented in numerical dimensions such as:

Good	—	—	—	—	—	—	—	Bad
	3	2	1	0	−1	−2	−3	

or can be presented on a descriptive dimension like that shown in Table 6.10 on p. 80. Numerical values can be assigned to the descriptive dimensions, and comparisons can be made between items of various groups in terms of mean scores.

Criteria for constructing a questionnaire

The characteristics of a good questionnaire can be summarised as follows (Wood, 1991; cited by Naoum and Coles, 1997, pp. 18–20):

1 It must deal with a topic of some significance that is important enough to the respondent to merit a response.
2 It must seek information not obtainable from other sources. You should not ask people to do your data gathering for you, especially when the data are readily available elsewhere.
3 It should be as short as possible but comprehensive enough to allow you to derive what you need without alienating the respondent.
4 It should be attractive in appearance, well laid out and well reproduced (see Appendix 2).
5 Where it contains directions they must be clear and complete.
6 Unless there is a very good reason for another format, questions should be arranged in categories which allow easy and accurate responses.
7 Questions must be as objective as possible without offering leading questions. For example, a question such as 'Do you not agree that site managers should have the right to have a say in finalising the building design?' is leading. Here, it might be difficult for site managers to answer 'No' in response to that question.
8 In their sequencing, questions should run from the general to the specific, from simple to complex, and from those that will create a favourable impression upon the respondent to those that may be sensitive.

Table 6.6 *The following statements are related to job satisfaction at work. Please indicate your reaction to each statement by ticking the appropriate cell*

Job satisfaction factors	Strongly agree	Agree	Neither agree nor disagree	Disagree	Strongly Disagree
1 Special wage increases should be given to employees who do their jobs well					
2 Better job descriptions would be helpful so that employees will know exactly what is expected of them					
3 Employees need to be reminded that their jobs are dependent on the company's ability to compete effectively					
4 Supervisors should give a good deal of attention to the physical working conditions of their employees					
5 Supervisors ought to work hard to develop a friendly atmosphere among their people					
6 Individual recognition for above-standard performance means a lot to employees					
7 Indifferent supervision can often bruise feelings					
8 Employees want to feel that their real skills and capacities are put to use in their jobs					
9 The company retirement benefits and share programmes are important factors in keeping employees in their jobs					
10 Almost every job can be made more stimulating and challenging					

11	Many employees want to give their best in everything they do			
12	Management could show more interest in the employees by sponsoring social events after hours			
13	Pride in one's work is actually an important reward			
14	Employees want to be able to think of themselves as the best at their own job			
15	The quality of the relationships in the informal work group is quite important			
16	Individual incentive bonuses would improve the performance of employees			
17	Visibility with upper management is important to employees			
18	Employees generally like to schedule their own work and to make job-related decisions with a minimum of supervision			
19	Job security is important to employees			
20	Having good equipment to work with is important to employees			

Source: Mullins (1996, pp. 514–516).

Table 6.7   *The following are a number of criteria which are commonly applied by clients of the building industry in assessing the performance of their projects. Please give a rating from 0 to 10 to each criterion according to the magnitude of importance each would be to your organisation (10 = very important)*

Criterion	Rating out of 10
1 Early start on site	
2 Reliability of the estimated design time	
3 Reliability of the estimated construction time	
4 Minimising the construction time	
5 Reliability of the estimated construction cost	
6 Obtaining a building at the cheapest cost	
7 Obtaining a building with low maintenance cost	
8 Obtaining a building with high aesthetic quality	
9 Obtaining a functional building to fit its purpose	
10 Input from the contractor related to buildability	
11 To have confidence in the contractor	

Table 6.8   *Would you please indicate, in priority order, which of the following factors you find important in being satisfied with your job. Please indicate which factor is first in importance, which is second, which is third and so forth (please circle the appropriate figure on the right-hand side)*

1	A well-paid job (having a good income and being able to afford the good things in life)	1 2 3 4 5 6 7 8
2	A prosperous job (having a good opportunity to develop myself)	1 2 3 4 5 6 7 8
3	An important job (a job full of achievement that brings me respect and recognition)	1 2 3 4 5 6 7 8
4	A secure job (making certain that I have steady work and steady wages)	1 2 3 4 5 6 7 8
5	Relationship with fellow workers (getting along well with the people I work with)	1 2 3 4 5 6 7 8
6	Relationship with superiors (getting along well with my supervisor)	1 2 3 4 5 6 7 8
7	Job interest (good chance to do work of my interest)	1 2 3 4 5 6 7 8
8	Working condition (working within a good physical job condition)	1 2 3 4 5 6 7 8

Table 6.9 *In your view, what are the most serious factors causing accidents on construction sites? (Please select not more than five and number them 1, 2, 3, 4, 5 in order of seriousness)*

_____ Age (very young or too old)	_____ Lack of experience to execute the task
_____ Lack of background safety training	_____ Paying operatives danger money
_____ Lack of personal care for safety	_____ Poor enforcement of safety laws and regulations
_____ Lack of safety training on site	_____ Bad supervisor's safety behaviour
_____ Bad workmates' safety behaviour	_____ Bad subcontractors' safety behaviour
_____ Mishandling of dangerous material	_____ Improper fixing of scaffolding
_____ Improper erection of steel	_____ Lack of inspection for safety
_____ Insufficient skill to operate plant	_____ Lack of provision of safety clothing
_____ Improper use of safety clothing	_____ Improper use of safety equipment
_____ Not issuing safety booklet	_____ Lack of trade union involvement
_____ Lack of site safety representative	_____ Lack of safety policy
_____ Lack of safety talk by management	_____ Not displaying safety posters
_____ Untidy site	_____ Badly planned and disorganised site

9 Bearing in mind point (8) above, you should avoid questions that may annoy or embarrass the respondent.
10 The questionnaire must provide for ease of tabulation and/or interpretation, and should be designed accordingly.

The above points illustrate the importance and the role of the questionnaire to the survey's success. The design of the questionnaire also requires careful attention, and consideration should be given to:

- Examining other questionnaires to identify possible clues.
- Obtaining as much help as possible in order to make sure it is easy to be understood by different audiences.

Table 6.10   *Think of your leader and describe him/her by completing the following scale. Place an 'X' in one of the eight spaces according to how well the adjective fits your leader. Look at the words at both ends of the line before placing your 'X'*

	8	7	6	5	4	3	2	1	
Pleasant	—	—	—	—	—	—	—	—	Unpleasant
Friendly	—	—	—	—	—	—	—	—	Unfriendly
Rejecting	—	—	—	—	—	—	—	—	Accepting
Helpful	—	—	—	—	—	—	—	—	Frustrating
Unenthusiastic	—	—	—	—	—	—	—	—	Enthusiastic
Tense	—	—	—	—	—	—	—	—	Relaxed
Distant	—	—	—	—	—	—	—	—	Close
Cold	—	—	—	—	—	—	—	—	Warm
Cooperative	—	—	—	—	—	—	—	—	Uncooperative
Supportive	—	—	—	—	—	—	—	—	Hostile
Boring	—	—	—	—	—	—	—	—	Interesting
Quarrelsome	—	—	—	—	—	—	—	—	Harmonious
Self-assured	—	—	—	—	—	—	—	—	Hesitant
Efficient	—	—	—	—	—	—	—	—	Inefficient
Gloomy	—	—	—	—	—	—	—	—	Cheerful
Open	—	—	—	—	—	—	—	—	Guarded

- Allowing for a pilot stage at the draft phase in order to get valuable responses and to detect areas of possible shortcomings.
- Close liaison with the supervisor and making sure that he/she has seen and approved the questionnaire.
- Trying different question orders at the pilot stage. This may assist in finding the best approach.
- Experimenting with different types of questions, both open and closed.
- Collecting the most relevant information and obtaining the maximum number of respondents by making sure that:
  - (a) You identify the sender and the person who receives the returned questionnaires.
  - (b) You know the purpose of the research and the questionnaire.
  - (c) There is an incentive for the respondent to complete the questionnaire.
  - (d) You reassure the respondent of the confidentiality of the questionnaire.
  - (e) You allow the respondent the opportunity to provide some personal insight not contained elsewhere.

Note to students: When trying to design the questionnaire, you need to ask your-self a number of questions such as:

- Are you using quantitative or qualitative measures?
- Is your study a comparative or a singular investigation?
- If it is a comparative study, how many survey groups are you investigating and who are they?
- How do the groups differ in their characteristics?
- What is the depth of the investigation? Is it a specific problem or a general-ised one?
- How many responses or cases do you need in order to answer your questions and achieve your objectives?
- If you are testing a theory, are you using control variables and why?

Once you have answered the above questions and designed the questionnaire, you can then invite the respondents to fill out the questionnaire or rate them or do whatever is required. It is absolutely essential to do a complete pilot study before you collect the final data for your main study.

A pilot study

Whenever you construct a questionnaire, it is advisable to complete a pilot study before you collect the final data from the whole sample. A pilot study provides a trial run for the questionnaire, which involves testing the wording of the question, identifying ambiguous questions, testing the technique that you use to collect the data, measuring the effectiveness of your standard invitation to respondents, and so on. Bell (1996, p. 84) described a pilot study as:

> getting the bugs out of the instrument (questionnaire) so that subjects in your main study will experience no difficulties in completing it and so that you can carry out a preliminary analysis to see whether the wording and format of questions will present any difficulties when the main data are analysed.

Bell (ibid.) went further and noted that you should ask your guinea pigs the fol-lowing questions:

1 How long did it take you to complete?
2 Were the instructions clear?
3 Were any of the questions unclear or ambiguous? If so, will you say which and why?
4 Did you object to answering any of the questions?
5 In your opinion, has any major topic been omitted?
6 Was the layout of the questionnaire clear/attractive?
7 Any comments?

You will probably be amazed by how much you will learn from a pilot study. The little extra time it takes to complete a pilot study test will be well spent.

Covering letter

After constructing your questionnaire, your next step is to write a covering letter to accompany your questionnaire. The letter should explain the purpose of the survey or questionnaire in order to encourage a high response. The content of the covering letter is particularly important in postal questionnaires because it is the only way you can persuade the subjects to respond to your questionnaire. Nachmias and Nachmias (1996, p. 20) write:

> A cover letter must succeed in overcoming any resistance or prejudice the respondent may have against the survey. It should (1) identify the sponsoring organization or the persons conducting the study, (2) explain the purpose of the study, (3) tell why it is important that the respondent answer the questionnaire, and (4) assure the respondent that the information provided will be held in strict confidence.

An example of a covering letter that can be used with a postal survey is presented in Figure 6.3.

Summary

Dear Sir/Madam

Re: Dissertation – BSc Construction Management

I am currently undertaking a Bachelor of Science Degree in Construction Management at London South Bank University. In fulfilment of this dissertation I am required to research a topic area and produce a dissertation. The topic I have chosen is 'Project Management as a Method of Building Procurement' and I am investigating the following aspects of its use:

1   The criteria which clients feel important in the selection of Project Management contracts.
2   The types of building for which Project Management is used and the dominant reasons for the selection of this type of procurement path for these buildings.
3   The types of clients who are predisposed to use Project Management.

I would be very grateful if you could complete the attached questionnaire and return it in the addressed, prepaid envelope provided. Needless to say, the information provided will be treated with strict confidence and individual firms will not be identified. Equally, a copy of the summary report will be available to the co-operating firms.

Yours faithfully,   Supervisor

Signature   Signature

Figure 6.3   *Example of postal survey covering letter.*

This chapter described the stages for constructing a questionnaire together with types and question formats. The foundation of all questionnaires, whether mailed or to be used for interviewing, is the questions. The principle that you need to follow in constructing your questionnaire is to go back to your dissertation proposal and start to ask specific questions related to the aim, objectives and hypothesis of your study.

Questions can be of two types: open ended and closed ended. Open-ended questions have the advantage of giving an opportunity to respondents to express their views on the subject but it can be rather difficult to analyse the results later. By contrast, closed-ended questions require a short response and their analysis is straightforward. However, you need to have sufficient knowledge on the subject of your investigation in order to offer respondents a set of response categories from which they should choose the one that most represents their opinions, views, attitudes or perceptions.

Questions can be either factual or an opinion type. Factual questions are designed to obtain objective data whereas opinion questions are designed to elicit subjective information. The questions can be formulated in various ways. The most common formats are checklist, grid, rating scale, Likert scale, numerical rating scale, ranking, and semantic differential scales. These formats are described in this chapter with examples. It is advisable to conduct a pilot study to test the wording of the questions, check the length of the questionnaire and make sure that the questions are not ambiguous. Finally, you need to write a covering letter to accompany your questionnaire stating who you are and the purpose of your study, ensuring confidentiality and perhaps offering an incentive to respond.

References

Bell, J. (1996) *Doing Your Research Project: A Guide for First-Time Researchers in Education and Social Science*. Open University Press.

Bell, J. (2005) *Doing Your Research Project: A Guide for First-Time Researchers in Education and Social Science*. Fourth edition. McGraw-Hill International.

Lazarsfeld, P. (1944) The controversy over detailed interviews: An offer for negotiation. *Public Opinion Quarterly*, 8: 38–60.

Moser, C. and Kalton, G. (1993) *Survey Methods in Social Investigation*. Dartmouth.

Mullins, L. (1996) *Management and Organizational Behaviour*. Pitman.

Mullins, L. (2010) *Management and Organizational Behaviour*. Pitman.

Nachmias, C. and Nachmias, D. (1996) *Research Methods in the Social Sciences*. Fifth edition. Arnold.

Naoum, S. and Coles, D. (1997) *Dissertation Guide: Instructions for Preparation, Control and Presentation of the Dissertation*. School of Construction, London South Bank University.

Oppenheim, A. (1996) *Questionnaire Design, Interviewing and Attitude Measurement*. Pinter.

Osgood, C.E. (1956) *Method and Theory in Experimental Psychology*. Oxford University Press.

Part III

Analysis and presentation of the results

7 Measurements and probability

Measurement is a procedure in which a researcher assigns numerals (numbers or other symbols) to empirical properties (variables) according to rules. It is closely linked to the research approach and questionnaire construction, which were discussed in Chapters 4 and 6 respectively. There are four levels of measurement: nominal, ordinal, interval and ratio. In some cases your research involves a search for a measure that is already developed and in other cases you need to design a measure. This chapter focuses on these levels of measurements in order to prepare the ground for the next exciting chapter: analysis of the results. This chapter also provides a statement of probability, which is an important term to understand in testing your research hypothesis. The contents of Chapter 7 are illustrated in Figure 7.1.

Note to students: The term 'measurement' is mainly used to quantify quantitative questions. I prefer to use the terms 'evaluation' and 'assessment' to process exploratory questions. Analysis of both quantitative and exploratory questions is discussed in Chapter 8.

Level of measurement

In order to be able to select the appropriate method of analysis, you need to understand the level of measurement. For each type of measurement, there is an appropriate method (or more than one) that can be applied and others that cannot.

Measurement is a procedure in which a researcher assigns numerals (numbers or other symbols) to empirical properties (variables) according to rules. Suppose you invited five contractors (A, B, C, D and E) to tender for building your project. Having found that the difference in price among five tenderers is minute, you decided to make the selection on the basis of which contractor best meets the following criteria: speed, quality and safety. These three criteria vary. For example, one contractor may deliver the project earlier and have a safety programme, but the quality of the finished product may be unsatisfactory. Accordingly, you decide to rank each of the three criteria on a scale 1 to 5, where 1 indicates total dissatisfaction and 5 stands for complete satisfaction. You then evaluate the five tenderers. After examining the scores, you may decide to appoint contractor B because it received the highest score on the three counts. The numbering process

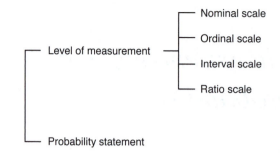

Figure 7.1   *Contents of Chapter 7.*

discussed above is a crude example of explaining the nature of measurement. However, it conveys the basic idea expressed in the definition of measurement, that is you assigned numerals to properties according to rules. The following section will explain the four principal levels of measurement, namely nominal, ordinal, interval and ratio. Your primary data collection should fall within one or more of these levels.

Nominal scale

Nominal numbering implies belonging to a classification or having a particular property and a label. It does not imply any idea of rank or priority. Nominal numbering is also conventional integers, that is positive and whole numbers (this may well be because most statistics are analysed by computer, which, as you know, handles numbers more easily than letters or strings). For example, if you conducted a survey to investigate the use of a particular project management software in the construction industry, you would count the number of companies using the package and categorise them as shown in Table 7.1.

The numbers given to the categories in Table 7.1 are nominal (i.e. name only). For example, number 1 (contractors) is not half of number 2 (architects) or in any way prior to or less than the others in quantity. The numbers are simply convenient but arbitrary labels for identifying each type of company. You could have used the label A instead of 1, B instead of 2, C instead of 3 and so on. The numbers within each category are called frequencies. The frequency distribution and the terms associated with it will be discussed in Chapter 8.

Table 7.1   *Categorisation table of companies using project management software*

Category				
1 (contractors)	2 (architects)	3 (quantity surveyors)	4 (engineers)	5 (others)
20	70	35	40	10

Ordinal scale

This is a ranking or a rating of data which normally uses integers in ascending or descending order. An example of an ordinal is when you ask an attitudinal question. For instance, you may want to measure your respondents' attitude to a motivational statement such as 'individual incentive bonuses would motivate people to work harder and in turn improve the performance of employees'. Here, the respondent is asked to mark a number representing his/her degree of agreement or disagreement with this statement. Table 7.2 illustrates a possible coding frame between the numbers and the answers. The numbers assigned to the agreement scale (5, 4, 3, 2, 1) do not indicate that the intervals between the scales are equal, nor do they indicate absolute quantities. They are merely numerical labels.

Another example of an ordinal scale is when respondents are asked to rank items by their own preference. For instance, if we asked eight people to rank the quality of a particular product in order of their preference, we might obtain Table 7.3.

Similarly to the previous example, the numbers in Table 7.3 do not indicate that the interval between the ranks are equal. Although the numbers are equally spaced, it does not imply that the property each represents is also equally spaced. If two respondents have the rank 8 and 6 and two others are ranked 7 and 5, it

Table 7.2 *Ordinal ranking scale*

	Strongly agree (5)	Agree (4)	Neutral (3)	Disagree (2)	Strongly disagree (1)
Site managers	4	3	5	5	0
Head office personnel	0	1	1	9	6
Operatives	7	5	4	1	0

Table 7.3 *Quality of product scores*

Person	Score	Rank of score
1	13	5.5
2	20	7
3	9	1
4	13	5.5
5	10	3
6	10	3
7	10	3
8	24	8

does not mean that the differences between the two pairs are equal. Notice the tied ranks in Table 7.3. In this example the score of 9 was given the first rank. As three people share the score of 10, you need to share the ranking, such as:

$$\frac{2+3+4}{3} = \frac{9}{3} = 3$$

For subjects 1 and 4 this means ranks 5 and 6 are shared, that is:

$$\frac{5+6}{2} = \frac{11}{2} = 5.5$$

Interval scale

The numbering system in the ordinal and nominal measurement is purely an arbitrary label for identifying each type of person. If you have a set of observations or data where the distance between each observation is constant, then this type of measurement is called an interval level of measurement. Often-used examples are minutes, kilograms, number of words recalled in a memory test and percentage marks in the exam. The interval between 20 and 30 minutes is the same as between 50 and 60 minutes. When it comes to numerical scores, such as numbers of items recalled per minute, you are dealing with numbers and you can assume that the distances between scores are the same. This type of measurement is another example of interval measurement because it assumes equal intervals between the data on a continuous scale.

Ratio scale

The ratio scale is similar to the interval scale except it involves the kind of numerical scale which has a natural zero, such as age, salary, time and distance. However, you do not need to bother about the difference between interval and ratio scales. For the level of statistics described in this book, both measurements are treated in exactly the same way.

Probability statement

The subject of probability is important to understand when you start to analyse your results. Statistical probability will tell you whether any differences in scores are due to your manipulation of the variables, as predicted by your research hypothesis or, alternatively, only due to chance fluctuations as stated in the null hypothesis. You do not need to be bothered now about the term 'null hypothesis'; it is discussed later, in Chapter 8.

We use the word 'probably' almost every day to express our views on certain things. Consider the following statements:

- It will probably rain next week.
- I will most probably visit my friend tomorrow.
- I will definitely pass my maths exam.

In the first statement you are giving a certain degree of chance that it will rain tomorrow. This chance is normally measured as a percentage out of 100. It could be 1 per cent, 5 per cent, 20 per cent, 50 per cent and so on. In the second statement you are making a more assured statement by saying 'most probably'. Again this could be any percentage out of 100, but rather towards the upper limit of the scale. It could be an 80 per cent, 90 per cent, 95 per cent chance and so on, but not 100 per cent. In the third statement you are making a more certain statement by using the word 'definitely' (i.e. 100 per cent). But on what basis have you made these statements or judgements? The second statement may be based on your experience, but the first and third statements are based on historical records. For example, your past record shows that you never failed the maths test in the past; hence, you are eliminating the chance of failing this time.

The term 'probability' can, therefore, be defined as the percentage that an event occurs in a number of times. In observational or experimental studies, if 1000 tosses of a coin result in 529 heads, the relative frequency of heads is $529/1000 = 0.529$. If another 1000 tosses result in 493 heads, the relative frequency in the total of 2000 tosses is $(529 + 493)/2000 = 0.511$. According to the statistical definitions, by continuing in this manner we should ultimately get closer and closer to a number which we call the probability of a head in a single toss of the coin. From results so far presented this should be 0.5 to one significant figure. To obtain more significant figures, further observations/experiments must be made.

Similarly, scientific and attitudinal research, related to the built environment, can be based on primarily probabilistic or indicative explanation. For example, a researcher might state that traditional contracts will most probably overrun on cost. His/her rationale is that, from past project records, in 8 out of 10 occasions the project exceeded the budget when using the traditional form of contract. But how significant is your result, that is how confident or sure are you of arriving at this concluding remark? The answer to this is: you have to apply statistical tests to determine the direction of your research. Chapter 8 provides details of the most popular statistical tests for the level of students reading this book.

Note to students: The statistical tests discussed in Chapter 8 will provide you with a probability that allows you to judge whether your results are significant or are due to chance. Later, you will find out that all the given examples will end up by stating the probability figure of the statistical test. For instance, you will come across an expression $P < 0.05$. This means that the probability of a result being due to chance is less than 5 per cent, or 5 in 100. Another, $P < 0.01$, means that the probability of a result being due to chance is less than 1 per cent, or 1 in 100, and so on. Therefore, the lower the probability figure the more confident you can be in concluding that there is a significant difference applied to your data.

The conventional level at which you can reject the null hypothesis and conclude that the results are significant is $P < 0.05$. Otherwise, the results of your test are not significant and you have to accept the null hypothesis of no relationship or association between the research variables.

Summary

This chapter discussed the level of data measurements and explained the term 'probability'. Measurement is a procedure in which you assign numerals (numbers or other symbols) to empirical properties (i.e. variables) according to rules. There are four levels of measurement and the data that you will collect should fall within one or more of these levels. The four levels are known as nominal, ordinal, interval and ratio. The nominal level implies belonging to a classification or having a label and does not imply any rank or priority. The ordinal level refers to data that are ranked or rated in ascending or descending order. The interval level is when you have a set of observations in which the distance between each observation is constant (e.g. minutes, kilograms and exam results). The ratio level is similar to the interval except it involves a natural zero.

The term 'probability' is defined as the percentage that an event occurs in a number of times. It is calculated to determine the direction of your study. The statistical tests that are explained in Chapter 8 will allow you to establish the confidence level of your research by testing the hypothesis. The probability figure, which is calculated using the statistical tests, will give you a level of significance by which you can judge whether to approve or disprove your research hypothesis.

8 *Analysis of the results*

Once you have collected the data, you will be ready to analyse the results to determine the direction of the study. You will be gathering a lot of information, which makes it difficult to present every bit of it. Therefore, it is expected that you give a summary of the data which highlights main trends and differences in the most appropriate manner. At this stage of your research study you will ask yourself a number of questions. For example, will I use a frequency distribution table or a bar chart to analyse each question in the questionnaire? Will I use a total score or should I analyse the data separately for each item in the questionnaire or rating scale? Which is the most appropriate test to use with the data: the *t*-test or the chi-square test? Should I compute some rank order correlation? Once you and your supervisor are satisfied with the answers to these questions, you can apply the statistics to find out if there are significant results.

This chapter describes, with examples, the methods of analysis that are commonly used to summarise and organise the data in a most effective and meaningful way. The chapter will cover the following:

- exploratory data analysis (open-ended questions);
- the descriptive method of analysis, including measurement of central tendency, the normal curve and the frequency distribution;
- the inferential statistical method of analysis, including the *t*-test, chi-square test, Spearman 'rho' ranking correlation and the product–moment correlation coefficient.

The contents of Chapter 8 are illustrated in Figure 8.1.

Exploratory data analysis (open-ended questions)

As discussed in Chapter 4, exploratory research is a type of qualitative research and can be described as a social or organisational behaviour research which produces results that are not obtained by statistical procedures or other methods of quantification. This type of data analysis refers to research about people's lives, their stories and behaviour, and it can also be used to examine organisations, relationships and social movements. Some of the data may be quantified afterwards, but the analysis is qualitative.

Figure 8.1 *Contents of Chapter 8.*

Research carried out in this way produces descriptive data such as people's own spoken or written words or observable behaviour. (Note that observational and experimental studies are not covered in this book.) The instrument or tool that is often used to collect exploratory research data is the open-ended type of questionnaire. The following section explains the procedure for processing open-ended questions.

Coding open-ended questions

Open-ended questions can be used in postal questionnaires as well as in interviews. The usual reason for using open-ended questions is that the researcher has no clear hypotheses regarding answers, which will be numerous and varied. Analysis of the open-ended questions can be rather complicated and not as straightforward as structured closed-ended questionnaires. It also requires a great skill to accurately report the information.

The best way to analyse open-ended questions is to code the information in terms of ideas and themes. The purpose of coding such questions is to reduce the large number of individual responses to a few general categories of answers that can be assigned a numerical code. In order to analyse open-ended questionnaires the following steps can be taken:

1 Place all similar answers in a general category and assign them a code. For example, individual clients asked about the use of construction management for their projects might give the following answers:
   (a) We build large and complex projects.
   (b) We want to have good control on the project.
   (c) It is quicker.
   (d) Construction management provides high integration.
   All of these answers can be categorised under 'favourable to construction management'.
      Other clients might give the following answers:
   (a) We build housing projects.
   (b) We are not sophisticated clients.
   (c) It is too risky.
   (d) It is not a straightforward process as with the JCT contract.
   All of these answers can be categorised under 'unfavourable to construction management'.
2 After establishing the general categories, you then need to divide them into, say, two to four sub-categories, and assign them a code. Coding is the process of identifying and classifying each answer with a numerical score or other character symbol. It usually involves entering the data for analysis or for computer storage. The coding categories should be exhaustive and provide for all possible responses. They should be mutually exclusive and independent so that there is no overlap among categories. On highly structured questionnaires, the categories may be pre-coded. With open-ended questions, the answers are post-coded. This means that the categories are assigned after the data have been collected. The categories must be assigned according to your judgement. It is better to assign too many categories than too few because it is easier to collapse several categories into one than to increase the number of categories (Zikmund, 1997).
      Table 8.1 shows an example of constructing categories and sub-categories to an open-ended question, and devising their coding scheme. These categories are for clients' responses to a question that asked for comments about the use of construction management for their projects.
3 After establishing the coding, choose the method of analysis which you think is suitable for your data (descriptive or/and inferential method). These methods are described later in this chapter. The suitability of each method depends on the nature of data, the type of measurement and your sample size.

Recording the information

Recording the information is an important step in the research process. Before starting any form of analysis you need to devise a data summary sheet for your data. The actual process of transferring the data from the questionnaire or data collection form (after the data have been collected) into a data summary form is

Table 8.1 *Example of coding open-ended questions*

Favourable to construction management

Sub-category 1 – Team relationship code

10 Smooth running project

11 Right attitude of team members

12 Contract of trust

13 High integration

14 Good communication

15

. . .

19 Other team relationship

Sub-category 2 – Project control code

20 High control on subcontractors

21 High control on safety

22 Good control on variations

23 Good control on quality

24

25

. . .

29 Other project control

Sub-category 3 – Project outcome code

31 Would not change the project objectives

32 High certainty on programme time

33 High certainty on project cost

34 Safer project

36

. . .

30 Other project outcome

Sub-category 4 – Miscellaneous code

41 Good for complex projects

42 Architects recommended

43 Concentrates on client needs

44 Would not cut corners

46

. . .

49 Other miscellaneous

Unfavourable to construction management

Sub-category 5 – Team relationship code

50 Too complicated

51 Does not eliminate 'them and us' attitude

52 Conflict with the professionals

53

54

. . .

59 Other team relationship

Sub-category 6 – Project control code

61 Difficult to control the programme

62 Does not control subcontractors

63 Difficult to control supervisors

64

65

. . .

69 Other project control

Sub-category 7 – Project outcome code

71 Expensive method

72 Not economical for small projects

73 Too risky to clients

74

75

. . .

79 Other project outcome

Sub-category 8 – Miscellaneous code

81 Do not like the concept

82 Use what our architect recommends

83 No universal accepted contract

84 The concept comes in different formats

85 Difficult to define and agree the work packages

. . .

89 Other miscellaneous

called the 'recording scheme' or 'production coding'. Table 8.2 is an example of a data summary form. (See also section 3 in Appendix 5: SPSS data entry.)

The first column of the data summary form is usually designated for the respondent's number. The rest of the columns represent the coded answers to the questions in the questionnaire. For example, question 1 in Table 8.2 may be an opinion question requiring the respondent to indicate strong agreement (coded 3), neither agreement nor disagreement (coded 2) or strong disagreement (coded 1). Question 2 may require a response of 'Yes' (coded 1) or 'No' (coded 2) and so on.

Notes to students

- The principle of the data summary form can be applied to open-ended questions (post-coded) as well as to closed-ended questions (pre-coded).
- The data summary form is usually inserted in the appendix of your dissertation because the data it includes are known as 'raw data'.

After recording the information, the field of statistics can be applied to the raw data so that some kind of interpretation and discussion can be made on the results. There are two methods you can use to analyse your data: the descriptive statistics method and the inferential statistics method (also known as bivariate statistical analysis). Both are explained below.

The descriptive statistics method

The descriptive statistics method is the simplest method of analysis, which provides a general overview of the results. It gives an idea of what is happening. The descriptive method will either analyse the responses in percentages (as in the case of a large sample) or contain actual numbers (as in the case of a small sample). In

Table 8.2   *Example of a data summary form (see also section 3 in Appendix 5: SPSS data entry)*

Respondent number	Question 1	Question 2	Question 3	Question 4 ...	Question 30
	Code number	Code number	Code number	Code number	Code number
	1 2 3	1 2	1 2 3	1 2 3	1 2 3
1	3	1	1	2	3
2	3	2	3	3	3
3	2	2	1	3	3
4	2	2	3	3	3
5	3	2	3	3	3
6	3	2	3	3	3
...					
37	1	2	2	1	2

this section I shall introduce three formal terms which are used to describe aspects of a group of data: these are 'frequency distribution', 'measurement of central tendency' and 'measurement of dispersion'.

Frequency distribution

When summarising large numbers of raw data it is often useful to distribute the data into categories or classes and to determine the number of individuals or cases belonging to each category. This is called 'category frequency'. It can be presented in the form of tabulation, a bar chart, a pie chart or a graph.

Tabulation

Tabulation is the simplest way to show the frequency of observations of each response to each variable under investigation. To conduct a frequency distribution you simply list the categories of the variable and count the number of observations in each. Table 8.3 shows the frequency distribution of the results related to 'an investigation of the marketing philosophy of private house-builders'. In this example, out of the 37 house-builders, eight respondents fall into category A and 29 respondents fall into category B. The frequencies can then be converted into percentages of the total number. Therefore, about 20 per cent of the house-builders believed that their firm's business philosophy is to 'first build the estate and then work out how best to sell the product' (i.e. category A), whereas 80 per cent believed that they 'first determine customers' wants and then design the product types and packages to satisfy those wants' (i.e. category B).

The other type of frequency is when two or more different categories of people respond to the questionnaire and the sample is small. For example, Table 8.4 shows results of clients' satisfaction on the performance of time of construction management contracts.

Notice that Table 8.4 shows only the actual frequencies with no percentages. It is important to use actual numbers when the sample is small as in the case of limited interviews. This is because a statement on the above figures, such as '80

Table 8.3   *Frequency distribution of marketing philosophy*

Question	No. of respondents in Category A:'We first build the estate and then work out how best to sell the product'	%	No. of respondents in Category B: 'We first determine customers' wants and then design the product'	%
In the house-building cycle, which action best describes your firm's business philosophy?	8	20	29	80

per cent of public clients were highly satisfied with the time of construction management', is factually accurate but can be misleading as the reader will assume a much larger total number of public clients than five.

Table 8.5 is an example of a frequency distribution applied for analysing secondary data collection. In this particular example, the data are the frequency of accidents record, published by the HSE, of 12 occupations.

Note to students: It is essential that, after presenting the results, you make comments on and interpretations of your findings. What do your findings tell you? What do they mean? Do they correspond closely with previous studies or not? Chapter 9 provides you with guidance on how to comment and interpret your results.

Table 8.4 *Level of clients' satisfaction on the performance of time of construction management contracts*

	High	Low	Total
Public clients (*n*=5)	4	1	5
Private clients (*n*=10)	7	3	10
Total	11	4	15

n, number of sample.

Table 8.5 *An example of a typical frequency distribution of injuries to employees in the construction industry for the based on secondary data gathered by the HSE's Field Operations Division (see raw data in Appendix 4)*

Worker occupation	No. of major accidents	%	No. of minor accidents	%
Bricklayer	72	4.0	550	5.9
Carpenter/joiner	136	7.5	1127	12.1
Electrician	108	6.0	330	3.5
Ground worker	58	3.2	139	1.5
Pavior	39	2.2	443	4.7
Scaffolder	62	3.5	222	2.4
Road worker	64	3.6	195	2.1
Driver	120	6.7	539	5.7
Labourer	316	17.6	1659	17.7
Maintenance	60	3.3	294	3.1
Manual production	104	5.8	548	5.8
Other	659	36.6	3329	35.5
Total	1798	100.0	9375	100.0

Bar charts/histograms

Horizontal or vertical bar charts can be used with the frequency distribution table or as an alternative method of presentation in the dissertation. Figure 8.2 is a bar chart for the data presented in Table 8.5. The variable 'worker occupation' is placed on the horizontal axis and the percentage frequency on the vertical axis. The actual frequencies are included at the top of the bars and the total frequency of $n=1798$ for major accidents and $n=9375$ for minor accidents is stated in the conventional format. The height of the bars indicates the proportion of the frequency.

Pie charts

Another method of presentation that is widely used is the pie chart. The areas of the pie chart represent the proportion of the respondents and are usually presented as percentages. Figure 8.3 is a pie chart representing the percentages of alternative contractual arrangements.

Note to students: The method of presentation chosen (tabulation, compound bar chart, component bar chart, graph or pie chart) depends on your judgement of which presentation is the clearest. Remember, always consult your supervisor.

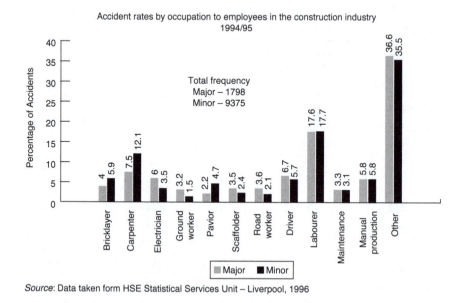

Source: Data taken form HSE Statistical Services Unit – Liverpool, 1996

Figure 8.2   *Example of a histogram presentation.*

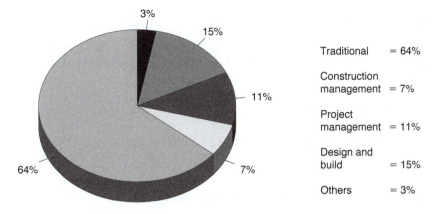

Figure 8.3   *Pie chart example representing the proportions of alternative con-tractual arrangements in the UK in 1996.*

Measurement of central tendency

This type of analysis is applied when you have a group of data and you wish to find the most typical value for the group, or the score which all other scores are evenly clustered around. These statistics are known as the 'mean', the 'median' and the 'mode'.

The mean

This is the average of all the values in a set of data. The mean is calculated by adding all the values in the group and then dividing by the number of values. Hence, the arithmetic mean of the cost per square metre of five contracts £564, £505, £556, £445 and £530 is taken as:

$$\frac{564+505+556+445+530}{5} = \frac{2600}{5} = £520$$

The median

The median of a set of numbers arranged in order of magnitude (i.e. in an array) is the middle value or the arithmetic mean of the two middle values. To establish the median you need to arrange the set of data in an array. Hence, the array of the above set of numbers is 445, 505, 530, 556, 564 and the median is, hence, 530.

The mode

The mode of a set of numbers is the value which occurs with the greatest frequency (i.e. the most common value). The mode may not exist, and if it does exist it may not be unique. For example:

1   The set 220, 220, 500, 700, 900, 900, 900, 1000, 1000, 1100, 1200 has mode 900.
2   The set 300, 500, 800, 1000, 1200, 1500, 1600 has no mode.
3   The set 200, 300, 400, 400, 400, 500, 500, 700, 700, 700, 900 has two modes, 400 and 700.

Measurement of dispersion based on the mean

This type of analysis can show you the degree by which numerical data tend to spread about an average value, known as 'variation' or 'dispersion'. This is represented by the formula:

$$\text{Mean deviation} = \frac{\Sigma\left(X - \bar{X}\right)}{N}$$

Hence, if the cost per square metre of five projects was taken and the results were £505.00, £557.00, £465.00, £458.00 and £530.00, the mean deviation can be calculated as follows:

Arithmetic mean = £503.00

$$\text{Mean deviation} = \frac{\begin{array}{c}|505 - 503| + |557 - 503| + |465 - 503| + \\ |458 - 503| + |530 - 503|\end{array}}{5}$$

$$= \frac{141}{5} = 28.2$$

Standard deviation

The standard deviation is another measure of the degree in which the data are spread around the mean. The theoretical basis of the standard deviation is complex and need not trouble the ordinary user (most scientific calculators have a function to calculate the standard deviation). However, a practical point to note is that the data should fall approximately into a so-called 'normal distribution'. When it does so the standard deviation provides a useful basis for interpreting the data in terms of probability (see 'Probability statement' in Chapter 7).

The formula for the standard deviation (SD) is:

$$SD = \sqrt{\frac{\sum (X - \bar{X})^2}{N}}$$

Hence, the SD for the five-unit cost is £35.70.

Normal distribution

Normal distribution is an important expression in the field of statistics because the selection of some inferential statistics depends on whether or not the data are normally distributed. The normal distribution curve can tell you a great deal about the scatter or distribution of the data (see Figure 8.4). The principal properties of the normal distribution curve are as follows (Nachmias and Nachmias, 1996):

* It is symmetrical and bell-shaped.
* The mode, the median and the mean coincide at the centre of the distribution.
* The curve is based on an infinite number of observations.
* A single mathematical formula describes how frequencies are related to the value of the variable.
* In any normal distribution, a fixed proportion of the observations lies between the mean and fixed units of the standard deviation. A range covered by one standard deviation above the mean and one deviation below it ($\bar{X} \pm 1SD$)

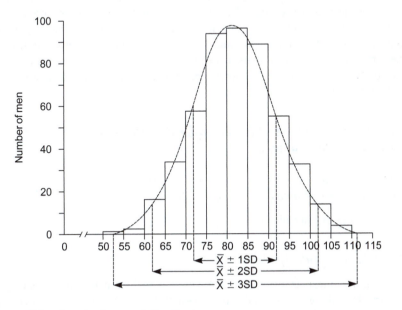

Figure 8.4   *A typical normal distribution curve.*

includes about 68 per cent of the observations. A range of 2 standard deviations above and 2 below ($\bar{X} \pm 2SD$) includes about 95 per cent of the observations. And a range of 3 standard deviations above and 3 below ($\bar{X} \pm 3SD$) includes about 99.73 per cent of the observations. Consequently, if you know the mean and standard deviation of a set of observations, you can obtain some useful information by simple arithmetic. By putting 1, 2 or 3 standard deviations above and below the mean you can estimate the ranges that would be expected to include about 68 per cent, 95 per cent and 99.7 per cent of the observations.

The inferential statistics method (also known as bivariate statistical analysis)

Many survey analyses entail the comparison of results for different parts of the sample, for example the proportion of traditional contracts that overrun on time versus the proportion of design and build contracts that overrun on time. In this case one might carry out a statistical significance test of the difference between the proportions. Statistical tests vary in their applications. Some tests are appropriate for testing differences in scores; other tests are suitable for assessing whether two sets of scores are correlated. For example, if you have two samples of normally distributed data and you want to find out whether there is a significant difference in the mean between the two samples, then you choose the *t*-test. If you have two or more categories of people and you want to find out whether there is significant difference in their attitude towards certain issues, then you use the chi-square test. If two groups of people are ranking a range of criteria and you want to know whether the differences in their ranking are significant, you will apply a ranking correlation (rho) and so on. The following sections will describe these tests in detail. Other statistical tests are also available but they are left for you to review. However, before describing these tests, there are five steps that you need to consider.

Steps to be carried out before and after the inferential (bivariate) statistical tests

Step 1: Formulate your research hypothesis in terms of the predicted results (like the one stated in your proposal)

See examples in Appendix 1.

Step 2: State the null hypothesis

The null hypothesis is a statement that you make which is the antithesis of your research hypotheses. It is usually an expression of no difference or no relationship between the variables. Suppose that the research hypothesis (H_1) states: 'Projects delivered under the traditional contracts are more expensive than similar projects delivered under the design and build contracts.' With the mean score for the cost of projects delivered under the traditional contracts designated as X_1 and in the design and build contracts as X_2, the research hypothesis, symbolised by H_1, will be:

$$H_1: X_1 > X_2$$

The null hypothesis, symbolised by H_0 will be:

$$H_0: X_1 = X_2$$

This means that your null hypothesis states: 'There is no significant difference in the mean cost between traditional contracts and the design and build contracts.' After applying the appropriate test you will find out whether your null hypothesis is true or false.

Step 3: Decide which test to use

Choose the appropriate statistical test for your data to determine the direction of your investigation. There are two main kinds of statistical tests that you can apply, known as 'parametric' and 'non-parametric' tests. A parametric test is a statistical test based on several assumptions about the parameters of the population from which the sample was drawn. To apply a parametric test, your data must comply with certain conditions. Among the most important conditions are the assumptions that the observations must be drawn from a normally distributed population and be of an interval scale (see discussion of normal distribution above) whereas a non-parametric test does not specify the normality condition. There are certain assumptions associated with most non-parametric tests; however, they are weaker than those associated with parametric tests. I will introduce the rationale, the rules and the steps to apply for each test as I go along.

When deciding the significance of your results also include tests for correlation. These kinds of tests measure the strength of the relationship between two or more variables and are usually applied on analytical studies. I will introduce the 'Spearman rank correlation' and 'Pearson product–moment correlation', as they are the most common tests and suitable for the level of students reading this book.

Step 4: Calculate and obtain the test statistics

After you decide on the test, you need to carry out the appropriate calculations on your research data. There are two ways in which you can carry out the calculations:

1 Manually.
2 Using a software package such as SPSS, Minitab or Statsmaster. These packages are easy to learn and, once you get the hang of using them, you will find it very easy to analyse your data in a matter of seconds. All you need to

do is to input your data from the data summary form (see Table 8.2) into the software spreadsheet and then select the appropriate statistics to carry out the calculations. Details of the SPSS package are described in this book on p. 121 and also in Appendix 5.

Step 5: Decide whether the result is significant (depending on significant level set)

Whichever type of statistical test you use, you will end up with a figure which is calculated in step 4 above. You then need to look in the statistical tables appropriate to that particular test to find out where your calculated figure falls. Each statistical table contains critical values against which the calculated figure can be compared. If your calculated figure is less than the critical value, then the results of your research are not significant and you should therefore accept your null hypothesis. If your calculated figure is equal to or more than the critical value in the statistical table, then the results of your research are significant; therefore reject the null hypothesis.

Appendix 3 gives four different statistical tables which correspond to the four statistical tests that will be described later. In certain statistical tables such as the *t*-distribution and the chi-square you will find the expression 'df'. This means 'degrees of freedom'. Degrees of freedom is a dimension that is used to find the critical value in the statistical tables. Sometimes it is determined by the number of subjects (respondents), sometimes by the number of subjects minus 1, and sometimes by the number of categories. However, you need not worry too much about the notion of degree of freedom or how to use the statistical tables. You will be guided on exactly what to do whenever degrees of freedom come up in connection with a statistical test.

There is one further point about the statistical inferential method and that is whether the research hypothesis is 'one tailed' or 'two tailed'. The point is that for a hypothesis which predicts a difference in only one direction (one tailed), there is a specified percentage probability that the difference might occur by chance but, if your research hypothesis makes a prediction that a difference might occur in either direction (two tailed), then there is double the probability that such differences might occur by chance. In the two-tailed condition there is the probability that a difference might occur in one direction plus the probability that a difference might occur in the other direction. However, you do not need to worry too much about the one-tailed and two-tailed notions; you can always use the probability level of the one-tailed direction.

Note to students: The statistical tests discussed below will provide you with a probability that allows you to judge whether your results are significant or are due to chance. Later, you will find out that all the worked examples will end up by stating the probability figure of the statistical test. For instance, you will come across the expression $P<0.05$. This means that the probability of a result being due to chance is less than 5 per cent, or 5 in 100. Another, $P<0.01$, means that the probability of a result being due to chance is less than 1 per cent, or 1 in 100, and so on. Therefore, the lower the probability figure the more confident you can be in concluding that there is a significant difference applicable to your data.

The conventional level by which you can reject the null hypothesis and conclude that the results are significant is $P<0.05$. Otherwise, the results of your test are not significant and you have to accept the null hypothesis of no relationship or association between the research variables or issues under investigation.

Parametric test (the t-test)

The *t*-test is a parametric test which is used to compare the difference between the mean scores of two samples.

Example

Table 8.6 gives results of the unit cost of two samples of projects completed over the same period of time and they were of a similar type. All projects were office blocks, reinforced concrete structure and of medium-sized projects, costing between £5 million and £10 million. However, one sample was taken from projects delivered using the design and build method of contracting and the other sample was taken from projects delivered using the traditional method of contracting. The aim of the research was to determine whether unit costs of Sample 1 (design and build projects) differ significantly from those of Sample 2 (traditional

Table 8.6 *Cost per square metre obtained from design and build projects and traditional projects*

Sample 1 (design and build projects) Unit cost (£) (X_1)	Sample 2 (traditional projects) Unit cost (£) (X_2)
564.00	505.00
521.00	557.00
445.00	465.00
560.00	458.00
480.00	530.00
540.00	480.00
585.00	665.00
426.00	525.00
530.00	605.00
475.00	495.00
$\bar{X}_1 = £512.60$	$\bar{X}_2 = £528.50$

projects). Following the directions given in the above section, the following steps were taken:

1 Formulate the research hypothesis: 'The unit cost of projects delivered under the traditional form of contract (X_1) is higher than similar projects delivered under the design and build contracts (X_2).' H_1 states that $X_1 > X_2$.

2 By implication, the null hypothesis is: 'There is no significant difference in the unit cost between the two samples.' H_0 states that $X_1 = X_2$.

3 The t-test is the most suitable test for this type of problem. The rationale for using this test is that:
   (a) The data are of an integer type (see definition in Chapter 7).
   (b) The problem is to compare the mean of two samples.
   (c) The samples are normally distributed. Note that, for the level of students reading this book, normality is not a strict condition.

4 Carry out the calculation (if not using the SPSS software package). In order for the mean unit cost of the two samples to be significant, the calculated value of t has to be equal or larger than the critical values of t given in Table A in Appendix 3. There are a number of formulas by which t can be calculated. This depends on whether the sample is small or large and whether it covers related or unrelated subjects. To simplify matters for students reading this book, t will be calculated by applying the following formula:

$$t = \frac{\bar{X}_1 - \bar{X}_2}{\sqrt{\frac{(SD_1)^2}{n_1} + \frac{(SD_2)^2}{n_2}}}$$

where

$\bar{X}_1$ = mean for sample 1	$\bar{X}_1 = 512.6$
$\bar{X}_2$ = mean for sample 2	$\bar{X}_2 = 528.5$
SD_1 = standard deviation for sample 1	$SD_1 = 50.8$
SD_2 = standard deviation for sample 2	$SD_2 = 61.9$
n_1 = number of subjects in sample 1	$n_1 = 10$
n_2 = number of subjects in sample 2	$n_2 = 10$

The standard deviation can be calculated using the formula given in the above section. However, most calculators can work out the SD in a matter of seconds so you can use one here. Therefore, in this example

$$t = \frac{512.6 - 528.5}{\sqrt{\frac{(50.8)^2}{10} + \frac{(61.9)^2}{10}}} = 0.63$$

5 Look up the significance of *t* in Table A of Appendix 3, taking into account the degrees of freedom, to see whether your result is significant.
For the *t*-test,

$$df = (n_1 - 1) + (n_2 - 1)$$
$$= (10 - 1) + (10 - 1) = 18$$

Look down the left-hand column of Table A to find the df (in this example 18). Then look along the row to see whether the calculated value of *t* is larger or equal to the critical values in the statistical table. In this example $t=0.63$, which is much smaller than the critical value of 2.10.

From the above findings, one can say that the null hypothesis (of no difference) has to be accepted and conclude that there is no significant difference in the unit cost between projects delivered using the design and build contracts and those using the traditional form of contracts.

Note to students: If the calculated value falls between two critical values in the statistical table, say $t=2.4$, you should use the expression $0.05 < P < 0.02$ for a one-tailed hypothesis.

Non-parametric test (the chi-square test)

The chi-square (symbolised as χ^2) is a test of association between two sets of data and can be used only when the data are nominal or ordinal. It predicts how many subjects in each group will fall into certain categories. Therefore, you have to test quite a number of subjects to make sure that a sufficient number of subjects turn out to be allocated to each category. Most statisticians consider 20 subjects to be the minimum number required in order to apply the chi-square test.

Example

This example is related to Proposal 1 in Appendix 1, that is to find out whether companies that performed well financially also had a business philosophy different from those that performed badly financially. Table 8.7 shows the data that were gathered from 37 companies. Financial performance was categorised as high (given numerate 2) or low (given numerate 1). The measurements of high and low were based on the annual profit of the companies. On the other hand, the business philosophy of each of the 37 companies was categorised as marketing oriented (given numerate 2) or production oriented (given numerate 1). The question at issue here is whether business philosophy and financial performance 'go' together or there is no association between the two variables. Following the direction given above, the following steps were taken.

Table 8.7   *Business philosophy and company performance*

Company	Business philosophy	Financial performance	Company	Business philosophy	Financial performance
1	1	2	20	1	2
2	2	2	21	2	2
3	1	2	22	2	1
4	2	2	23	2	2
5	1	2	24	1	1
6	2	2	25	1	1
7	1	1	26	1	1
8	2	1	27	2	1
9	2	2	28	2	2
10	2	2	29	1	1
11	2	2	30	1	1
12	2	2	31	1	1
13	1	2	32	1	1
14	2	2	33	2	2
15	2	2	34	1	1
16	2	2	35	2	2
17	2	1	36	2	1
18	2	1	37	2	2
19	2	2			

1 Formulate the research hypothesis: 'The type of business philosophy can have an effect on the financial performance of the private house-builders.'

2 By implication the null hypothesis is: 'The financial performance of private house-builders that have a marketing-oriented philosophy does not differ from those that have a production-oriented philosophy.'

3 The chi-square test is appropriate to this kind of problem. The rationale for using this test is that:
   (a) The data are nominal (see definition in Chapter 7).
   (b) The research subjects (private house-builders) can be allocated into categories. In this example there are two categories.
   (c) The sample is quite large (37 subjects).

4 Carry out the calculation (if not using a computer). In order for the financial performance of the two categories to differ significantly, the calculated value of χ^2 has to be equal to or larger than the critical values of χ^2 given in Table B of Appendix 3. To calculate χ^2 manually you need to take the following steps:

(a) From the data summary sheet in Table 8.6, allocate the replies into one of the two categories, high financial performance or low financial performance. The results are shown in the form of a 2×2 table known as a 'contingency' table. The cells representing each of the categories are numbered 1 to 4 in Table 8.8. Remember that the figures in the table represent the number of subjects that fall into each category; they are not scores or percentages. For example, in the first top right cell, the number 6 means that in the sample there are six companies that performed low financially and also have a marketing-oriented philosophy (check the rest by yourself).

Note to students: The rationale of the chi-square test is that it compares the 'observed' frequencies (O) in each of the squares (cells) of the contingency table with the 'expected' frequencies (E) for each cell if the differences are due to chance, as stated in the null hypothesis. In other words, the test compares the actual numbers of subjects (private house-builders) that fall into each cell as against the numbers of subjects we would expect to fall into each cell if there were in fact no differences between the financial performance of the two types of subjects (i.e. the marketing-oriented companies and the production-oriented companies). The observed frequencies are already known from the investigation (as shown in Table 8.8). Therefore, the expected frequencies need to be calculated. If the observed frequencies are close to the expected frequency, then the results are not significant. However, if the differences between the observed frequency and the expected frequencies are large, then the research hypothesis is supported. Therefore, the larger χ^2, the more significant are the results, so the computed value of χ^2 should be equal or larger than the critical values in Table B of Appendix 3.

(b) To calculate the expected frequency (E) for each cell, follow the procedure below:
   (i) Add the total observed frequencies for the rows and columns. In this example, they are equal to 23, 14, 22, 15. Here, the grand total is 37 $(23 + 14$ for rows) and $(22 + 15$ for columns) – see Table 8.8.
   (ii) Multiply the two relevant marginal totals for each cell and divide by the total number of subjects N.
   Therefore,

   for Cell 1: the expected frequency $(E) = 22 \times 23/37 = 13.67$
   Cell 2: $E = 15 \times 23/37 = 9.32$
   Cell 3: $E = 22 \times 14/37 = 8.32$
   Cell 4: $E = 15 \times 14/37 = 5.67$

   (iii) Find the value of chi-square from the formula $\chi^2 = \sum (O - E)^2 / E$, where
   O = observed frequencies for each cell (as shown in Table 8.8)
   E = expected frequencies for each cell (as calculated above)
   Σ = add up the results of $(O - E)^2/E$ calculated for each cell.

Table 8.8 *Contingency table between business philosophy and financial performance*

	High financial performance (2)	Low financial performance (1)	Total
	1	2	
Marketing oriented (2)	17	6	23
	$E=$ 13.67	$E=$ 9.32	
	3	4	
Production oriented (1)	5	9	14
	$E=$ 8.32	$E=$ 5.67	
Total	22	15	37

Chi-square$=5.26$.

Therefore,

$$\chi^2 = \frac{(17-13.67)^2}{13.67} + \frac{(6-9.32)^2}{9.32} + \frac{(5-8.32)^2}{8.32} + \frac{(9-5.67)^2}{5.67}$$
$$= 0.81+1.18+1.32+1.95 = 5.26$$

5 Look up the significance of χ^2 in Table B of Appendix 3, taking into account degrees of freedom, to see whether your result is significant.

6 For the χ^2, the degree of freedom (df)$=(r-1)(c-1)$, where
  $r=$number or rows in contingency Table 8.8 ($r=2$)
  $c=$number of columns in contingency Table 8.8 ($c=2$)
  Therefore, df$=(2-1)(2-1)=1$

Table B gives critical values against which the calculated value of χ^2 can be compared. The level of significance depends on the degrees of freedom (df). In this example, df$=1$ so we should look along that row in Table B. Since our calculated value of χ^2 is 5.26 and so is larger than the critical value of 3.84 for $P<0.05$, the results of this research are significant.

From the above finding one can say that the null hypothesis (of no difference) has to be rejected and conclude that there is a significant difference in the financial performance between house-builders that had a marketing-oriented philosophy and those that had a production-oriented philosophy.

Notes to students

- In this example, the calculated value of χ^2 falls between two critical values in the statistical table (between 0.05 and 0.02). In this case we use the expression $0.02 < P < 0.05$.
- Remember, it is absolutely essential to make comments on and interpretations of your findings after the analysis. What do your findings tell you? What do they mean? Do they correspond closely with previous studies or not? Chapter 9 provides you with guidance on how to comment and interpret your results.

Spearman rank correlation coefficient

The Spearman rho correlation is a non-parametric test for measuring the difference in ranking between two groups of respondents scoring a number of issues, attributes or factors. The test can be applied when:

- The question is requesting a ranking value like that on pp. 78–80.
- The question is requesting a scoring value and the scores are then converted into rankings like that in Table 6.7 on p. 78.
- The question is requesting rating values and the ratings are converted into rankings those in Table 6.3 on p. 73 and Table 6.6 on p. 76.

Example 1

Consider the question in Table 68 on p. 78. The researcher sent the questionnaire to site operatives of two different industries: to 50 workers in Indonesia and to 50 workers in the UK. The student wanted to find out whether there is a difference in attitude between the two groups towards the factors that can affect job satisfaction. Forty-two replies were received from UK workers and 44 replies from Indonesian workers. Table 8.9 shows the data obtained. Column 1 represents the average rank for UK workers and column 2 represents the average rank for the Indonesian workers. Columns 3 and 4 represent the difference in ranks and their squares respectively. The following steps were taken to apply the appropriate test:

1 Formulate the research hypothesis: 'The factors that satisfy workers with their jobs differ between Indonesian workers and UK workers.'
2 By implication, the null hypothesis is: 'There is no significant difference in the ranking of job satisfaction factors between the two industries.'
3 The Spearman rank correlation is an appropriate test for this type of problem. The rationale for using this test is that:
   (a) The attitude is measured on an ordinal scale (see definition in Chapter 7).

Table 8.9   *Average ranking of UK workers and Indonesian workers to factors influencing job satisfaction*

Job satisfaction factor	UK ranks (1)	Indonesia ranks (2)	di (3)	di² (4)
1 A well-paid job (having a good income and being able to afford the good things in life)	3	1	2	4
2 A prosperous job (having a good opportunity to develop myself)	1	5	4	16
3 An important job (a job full of achievement that brings me respect and recognition)	4	7	3	9
4 A secure job (making certain that I have steady work and steady wages)	2	2	0	0
5 Relationship with fellow workers (getting along well with the people I work with)	8	6	2	4
6 Relationship with superiors (getting along well with my supervisor)	6	4	2	4
7 Job interest (good chance to do work of my interest)	5	3	2	4
8 Working condition (working within a good physical job condition)	3	8	5	25
Total di²				66

(b)   The problem is to measure the amount and significance of a correlation between people's rank on a number of issues.

4   Carry out the calculation (if not using a computer). Here, the prediction is that, if there is a high positive correlation in opinions between the two groups, then the low ranking of one item by the UK operatives should correspond to low ranking by operatives in Indonesia and vice versa. However, if there is no correlation (as stated by the null hypothesis) the average ranks will be mixed up since one group could have a high ranking on the eight-point scale whereas the other may have a low ranking for the same item. To calculate rho you need to apply the following simple formula:

$$\rho = 1 - \frac{6 \sum d_i^2}{N\left(N^2 - 1\right)}$$

where di = the difference in ranking between each pair of factors
N = number of factors

Therefore, in this example,

$$\rho = 1 - \frac{6(66)}{6(64-1)}$$

$$= 1 - \frac{396}{504} = 0.21$$

5 Look up the significance of rho in Table C of Appendix 3, the calculated rho value of 0.21 against the value N (number of factors); in our example $N=8$, is less than the critical value of 0.643 for $p<0.05$ in the one-tailed test. Therefore, you can conclude that there is no correlation between the attitudes of the two groups, and the null hypothesis should be accepted. This means that most of the factors that are considered very important to satisfy the UK worker are less important to workers in Indonesia and vice versa.

Note to students: The value of N will be taken as 'number of subjects' if the question or the investigation is of a different format, as in the case of an experimental study. In construction, an example could be when 30 people are asked to rate two different attributes; N will be calculated as the number of subjects that took part in the research, which, in this case, is 30 (see example in section 9.3 of Green and D'Oliveirs's 1993 book).

Example 2

In this example I will discuss a situation when the question is requesting a rating value and the ratings are converted into ranks. Here, the student asked two groups of people, namely head office personnel and site managers, to respond to a number of questions by ticking their opinions on a three-point scale. Thirty-six fully completed questionnaires were returned, 19 from contract managers working at head office and 17 from experienced site managers. After receiving the data and recording the information in the data summary sheet, the student assigned scores to the ratings. Highly important=3 points, moderately important=2, and less important=1. Table 8.10 shows results of the survey. Here, the student applied a simple arithmetic to convert the average ratings into percentages of actual scores. Hence, Table 8.10 was constructed calculating the maximum possible scores, actual scores and percentage of actual scores for head office respondents and site managers. The maximum possible score for each factor relating to head office respondents is $3 \times 19 = 57$ and for site managers is $3 \times 17 = 51$. For example, 10 of the head office personnel thought that 'project planning' can highly affect productivity, eight thought moderately and one did not think it has any effect at all.

Table 8.10 *Ranking of head office personnel and site managers to factors influencing site productivity*

Productivity factor	Head office actual scores (%)	Rank (A)	Site managers actual scores (%)	Rank (B)	di (A−B)	di²
1 Delegation of responsibilities	58	24	70	14.5	9.5	90.2
2 Integration of information	77	5	83	3	2.0	4.0
3 Project planning	82	1	85	1	0	0
4 Scheduling of project activities	75	9	75	14.5	5.5	30.2
5 Level of authority	53	27.5	52	29	1.5	2.2
6 Supervision of subordinate	75	9	73	11	2.0	4.0
7 Communication	60	22	78	8.5	13.5	182.0
8 Senior managers' role in contract meetings	75	9	73	11	2.0	4.0
9 Attitude of site personnel	75	9	64	20	11.0	121.0
10 The decision-making process	75	9	64	20	11.0	121.0
11 Procurement of materials	77	5	83	3	2.0	4.0
12 Site programme	77	5	78	8.5	3.5	12.2
13 Accuracy of technical information	67	14.5	81	6	8.5	72.2
14 Fitness of tools for tasks	67	14.5	70	14.5	0	0
15 Knowledge of technology	67	14.5	81	6	8.5	72.2

No.						d_i^2
16	Interference on workmanship	67	14.5	73	11	3.5	12.2
17	Site layout	63	20.5	62	24.5	4.0	16.0
18	Promotion of employee	53	27.5	64	20	7.5	56.2
19	Resentment of company policy	65	18	64	20	2.0	4.0
20	Incentive for good performance	55	26	62	24.5	1.5	2.5
21	Opportunities to exercise skill	39	29	68	17	12.0	144.0
22	Response to employee grievances	58	24	62	24	0	0
23	Uncertainty about career	72	12	70	14.5	2.5	6.25
24	Work environment	81	2	83	3	1.0	1.0
25	Experience of employees	79	3	81	6	3.0	9.0
26	Contract administration skill	65	18	64	20	2.0	4.0
27	Knowledge of techniques	63	20.5	62	24.5	4.0	16.0
28	Training on new technology	58	24	59	27.5	3.5	12.2
29	Availability of skilled personnel	65	18	59	27.5	9.5	90.2
	Total d_i^2						1092.7

Note: $\rho = 1 - \dfrac{6\sum d_i^2}{N(N^2-1)} = 1 - \dfrac{6 \times 1092.7}{29(841-1)} = 0.73$, hence, $P < 0.005$

The actual scores of head office personnel to 'project planning' have then been calculated as:

$$(10 \times 3) + (8 \times 2) + (1 \times 1) = 47$$

Therefore, the percentage of maximum scores was

$$47/57 \times 100 = 82 \text{ per cent}$$

Table 8.10 shows the complete results. The ranking of the 29 factors between the two groups was tested using Spearman's rho, with the correlation found to be significant at $P < 0.005$ (see calculation for rho $= 0.73$ in the note to Table 8.10). This indicates that high ranking for one productivity factor by one sample, in most cases, corresponds to high ranking by the other sample and vice versa. The research hypothesis, therefore, can be rejected, and the null hypothesis can be accepted, concluding that the difference in opinion between head office personnel and site managers towards factors influencing productivity is not significant.

Pearson product–moment correlation coefficient

The correlation coefficient (r) is a parametric test which is used when you have two sets of scores and you want to calculate whether there is a strong relationship between them. Whereas the Spearman test can be used with any data, the Pearson requires the research data to be measured on an 'interval' scale and to meet the other assumptions for parametric tests. With the Pearson correlation, the relationship can be either positive or negative and the strength of the relationship is measured on a scale that varies from $+1$ through 0 to -1. When one variable increases as the other increases the correlation is positive; when one decreases as the other increases it is negative. The variable can be either factual or perceptual. For example, we would say that the speed of construction is correlated with the unit cost of the building. Since one increases with the other the correlation is called positive. In contrast there is a negative correlation between complexity of the building and speed of construction. In other words, the more complex the project, the slower the rate of construction.

After you collect the data, it is best to draw a scatter diagram, which is a graph with axes X and Y corresponding to the two variables being measured. The two variables can represent two dependent factors, two independent factors, or one dependent factor and one independent factor. The scatter diagram should show at a glance whether or not a relationship is likely to exist. Figure 8.5 shows a number of examples.

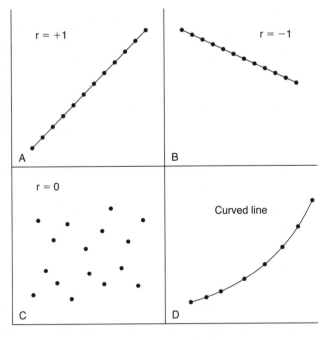

Figure 8.5 *Examples of correlation scatter diagrams.*

Example 1 of Pearson correlation coefficient (manual calculation)

Let us assume that Table 8.11 is a set of data collected by the researcher and he/she wants to assess whether there appears to be a correlation between the two measurements labelled X and Y. For instance, X could be the mathematics marks of the students out of 100 per cent, Y could be the physics marks out of 100 per cent. The question at issue is to find out whether maths performance and being good at physics 'go' together or there is no connection between the two kinds of ability.

In order to calculate the significance of the correlation, the following steps should be taken:

1 Formulate the research hypothesis: 'Students who are good at maths are also good at physics, students who are average at maths are also average at physics and students who are poor at maths are also poor at physics.'
2 By implication, the null hypothesis is: 'There is no significant relationship between the maths results and physics results.'
3 The Pearson product–moment correlation is an appropriate test to apply. The rationale for using this test is that:
    (a) The data are of an interval type (see definition in Chapter 7).
    (b) The problem is to establish a relationship between two variables.

Table 8.11   *Scores on variables X and Y for 12 subjects*

Number of subject	Variable X	Variable Y	$(X) \times (Y)$	X^2	Y^2
1	65	68	4420	4225	4624
2	63	66	4158	3969	4356
3	67	68	4556	4489	4624
4	64	55	3520	4096	3025
5	68	69	4692	4624	4761
6	62	66	4092	3844	4356
7	70	68	4760	4900	4624
8	66	65	4290	4356	4225
9	68	71	4828	4624	5041
10	67	67	4489	4489	4489
11	69	68	4692	4761	4624
12	71	70	4970	5041	4900
Total	800	801	53467	53418	53649

(c) The sample is normally distributed. Note that, for the level of students reading this book, normality is not a strict condition.

4 Carry out the calculation of the correlation coefficient (if not using the computer). In order for the scores for the two variables to be highly correlated, the calculated value of r has to be equal or larger than the critical values of r given in Table D in Appendix 3. The correlation coefficient (r) can be calculated from the following formula:

$$r = \frac{N\sum XY - \sum X \sum Y}{\sqrt{\left[N\sum X^2 - \left(\sum X\right)^2\right]\left[N\sum Y^2 - \left(\sum Y\right)^2\right]}}$$

$r = 0.59$

5 Looking up the significance of r in Table D of Appendix 3, the correlation coefficient of 0.59 indicates a positive correlation between variable X (maths marks) and variable Y (physics). Looking up for significance in Table D of Appendix 3, for df$=(10-2)$, the calculated value of 0.59 exceeds the critical value 0.5494 for $P<0.05$ (one tailed) and therefore the researcher can conclude that there is a significant relationship between the two variables. This means that there is less than 5 per cent probability that it was due to a chance distribution of scores. However, in interpreting correlation it is important to remember that 'correlation is not causation'. There may or may not be a causal

connection between the two correlated variables. However, for the level of students reading this book, it will be enough to comment on what was stated in your research hypothesis. In this example, you can say that the research hypothesis is valid and, therefore, reject the null hypothesis, concluding that 'Students who perform well in maths also perform well in physics.' If your dissertation contains a number of findings such as these, then it can be said that your dissertation has substance.

Data analysis using the SPSS (Statistical Package for the Social Sciences) software

SPSS is one of the most widely used statistics analysis packages in providing detailed and comprehensive statistics analysis on various types of data. It can perform all of the statistical tests discussed in this chapter: the *t*-test, chi-square test, Pearson correlation coefficient, ranking correlation, regression analysis and many more tests of significance. The spreadsheet-like interface allows users to enter data easily and to conduct in-depth data analysis.

SPSS is often used in research as a tool to analyse survey/questionnaire feedback. Although the graphics output may not have the level of customisation offered by Excel, it is often used in conjunction with Excel to provide full statistical analyses and professional presentation of data in research reports and dissertations.

Appendix 5 gives a full explanation of the SPSS package.

Worked example of Pearson correlation coefficient (calculated using the SPSS package)

This example is based on research that was conducted at London South Bank University by Tim Whitworth in 2010; the result was later published in the 6th International Structural Engineering and Construction Conference (ISECC-6) in Zurich, 21–26 June 2011 (see Naoum *et al.*, 2011).

Title of research

Is there a relationship between the lean concept and productivity rate of construction projects?

Aim

To demonstrate in a graphical format the relationship between implementing a lean management initiative and productivity rate of construction projects.

Brief research methodology

Data were collected from 37 randomly selected construction projects across commercial, residential, retail, industrial, health and education sectors through project managers/directors who were members of the Chartered Institute of Building.

Respondents were asked to select answers to 37 questions, which translate into scoring of between 0 (no leanness) and 4 (total leanness). The questions were grouped under nine areas of leanness identified by Taj (2008): project activities, team approach, processes, maintenance, layout, supply chain, start-ups, quality and schedule. An average leanness in terms of percentage is calculated for each area and the final project leanness is assessed based on the average of leanness score for all nine areas, in the same way as computed by Taj (2008) in lean assessment.

Productivity-related data for each project were collected from the same respondents in order to compute the productivity level for a project. In this research, productivity is defined as the output quantity with respect to the input quantity, which is evaluated as the gross floor area (m^2) constructed per week divided by the number of workers involved.

Result

The leanness and productivity scores for all 37 projects are shown in Table 8.12.

Table 8.12   *Construction leanness scores and productivity data*

Project no.	Leanness score (%)	Productivity (m^2/man week)
1	39.0	0.21
2	80.6	0.74
3	37.5	0.13
4	35.1	0.14
5	37.3	0.22
6	66.1	0.24
7	60.9	0.51
8	71.0	0.64
9	35.4	0.10
10	60.4	0.53
11	50.0	0.33
12	79.9	1.23
13	70.2	0.63
14	38.8	0.24
15	49.9	0.22
16	80.0	0.83

17	74.7	0.61
18	44.7	0.31
19	43.6	0.13
20	39.7	0.22
21	56.9	0.44
22	28.0	0.21
23	31.9	0.20
24	39.9	0.23
25	82.6	0.94
26	53.4	0.41
27	39.4	0.21
28	42.3	0.23
29	72.7	0.91
30	91.6	1.22
31	54.7	0.30
32	11.0	0.01
33	35.8	0.22
34	25.3	0.12
35	72.9	0.62
36	86.0	0.84
37	60.5	0.43

Calculating the strength of the relationship using the SPSS package

In order to calculate the significance of the correlation, the following steps were taken:

1 The research hypothesis: 'Projects that implement lean management initiatives will result in a higher rate of productivity on site.'
2 The null hypothesis is: 'There is no significant relationship between lean construction and productivity rate.'
3 The Pearson product–moment correlation is an appropriate test to apply. The rationale for using this test is the same as in Example 1 above.
4 Carry out the calculation of the correlation coefficient using the SPSS package as shown in Appendix 5.

Figure 8.6 presents the scatter plot of productivity and leanness for all 37 projects. Pearson correlation analysis shows that there is a strong positive linear relationship between leanness and productivity with $r=0.91$ ($P<0.005$).

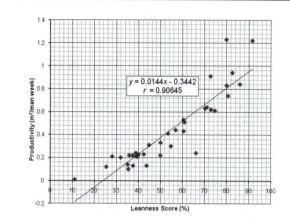

Figure 8.6 *Regression analysis and Pearson product–moment correlation coefficient.*

The result signifies a less than 0.5 per cent probability that the relationship was due to a chance distribution of scores. For the purpose of this study the research hypothesis is proven to be valid, and therefore the null hypothesis can be rejected.

Statistics of the 37 projects were compared with those derived from the manufacturing projects in Taj's study (2008). The leanness score for the 65 manufacturing projects in Taj's research yielded an average score of 55.3 per cent. This represents a moderate level of leanness overall for the manufacturing sector. The expectation that the construction industry is not far behind is evident, as a mean leanness score of 53.5 per cent is obtained from this study. A two-tailed, independent-sampled t-test was conducted using SPSS to test the hypothesis that there is no significant difference between the mean leanness scores of manufacturing and construction projects. Levene's test of equality of variances shows that $F = 16.6$ is significant ($p < 0.05$) and results from the 'equal variances not assumed' section are used in the comparison of means. A t-value of 0.49 at $P = 0.63$ indicates there is no significant difference between the mean leanness score of construction projects surveyed in this research and that of the manufacturing projects in Taj's study.

Concluding comments of this worked example

Although the focus of construction is heading in the same direction as manufacturing, literature is more advanced in the manufacturing industry. With the trend proving the same and no assessment tool available in the construction industry, the review highlighted that it is viable to transfer the same methodology. In hindsight, more research needs to be carried out in the construction industry in order to investigate in more detail the key assessment areas of lean in construction rather than adapting manufacturing ones.

The research sample provided the study with a broad scope of project, size, type and cost, which resulted in varying degrees of productivity output. The data proved conclusively that there is a strong relationship between a high lean implementation and high productivity on UK construction sites. The results proved that the probability of a result being due to chance is less than 0.5 per cent, which proves that there is a significant relationship between the two variables.

Summary

This chapter explained the methods by which you can analyse the results of your investigation. It explained first the descriptive method and then the inferential method with worked examples.

The descriptive method of analysis includes the frequency distribution, measurement of central tendency and measurement of dispersion. With the descriptive method you can apply a straightforward calculation to show how the respondents are distributed on all the items of the investigation. For example, 20 per cent of the house-builders believed that their firm's business philosophy is to 'first build the estate and then work out how best to sell the product', whereas 80 per cent believed the opposite. Such breakdowns of percentages or the numbers of observations that fall into each of several categories are termed 'frequency distribution'. The frequency distribution can be illustrated in a table, bar chart, graph or pie chart, all of which are demonstrated in this chapter.

Measures of central tendency are applied when you have a group of data and you wish to find the most typical value for the group or the score which all other scores are evenly clustered around. These statistics are known as the mean, mode and median.

Measurement of dispersion is a type of analysis that can show you the degree by which numerical data tend to spread about an average value. This spreading is called variation, dispersion or standard deviation.

The inferential method of analysis concentrates on the nature of the relationship between two variables and on the construction of measures of relationship. Four types of tests were explained with examples in this chapter: t-test, chi-square test, Spearman (rho) ranking correlation and Pearson product–moment correlation (r).

The t-test is a parametric test and it is appropriate for use when you want to compare the difference between the mean scores of two groups of data. The data have to be of interval type and normally distributed, and can be used, for example, to find out if there is a significant difference in the unit cost between two types of contracts.

The chi-square test is a test of association between two sets of data and can be used when the data are nominal or ordinal. It predicts how many subjects in each group fall into certain categories, for example how many companies that are marketing oriented also have high financial performance, and how many product-oriented companies also perform poorly financially.

Spearman's ranking correlation (rho) is a non-parametric test for measuring the difference in ranking between two groups of respondents, scoring a number of issues, attitudes or factors. It can be used, for example, to find out how two groups of people, say managers and operatives, rank their priorities against a list of job satisfaction factors. The question at issue here is whether there is a significant difference in their rankings.

The Pearson product–moment correlation (r) is a test used when you have two sets of data and you want to calculate whether there is a strong relationship between them. The relationship can be either positive or negative and the strength of it is measured on a scale that varies from +1 through 0 to −1. For example, it can be used to find out whether speed of construction is related to size of project.

References and additional reading

Bell, J. (2005) *Doing Your Research Project: A Guide for First-Time Researchers in Education and Social Science*. Fourth edition. McGraw-Hill International.

Coolican, H. (1993) *Research Methods and Statistics in Psychology*. Hodder and Stoughton.

Green, J. and D'Oliveirs, M. (1993) *Learning to Use Statistical Tests in Psychology: A Student's Guide*. Open University Press.

Kennedy, J. and Neville, A. (1976) *Basic Statistical Methods for Engineers and Scientist*. Second edition. Harper and Row.

Naoum S., Whitworth, T. and Fong, D. (2011) 'Is there a relationship between the lean concept and productivity rate of construction projects?', 6th International Structural Engineering and Construction Conference (ISEC – 6), 21–26 June, Zurich. Paper ID S1-C33.

Nachmias, C. and Nachmias, D. (1996) *Research Methods in the Social Sciences*. Fifth edition. Arnold.

Rassam, F. (1989) 'Marketing profile and financial performance of private house building companies', MSc dissertation, Bath University.

Siegel, M. (1995) *Theory and Problems of Statistics*. Schaum's Outline Series, McGraw-Hill.

Swinscow, T. (1987) *Statistics at Square One*. British Medical Association.

Taj, S. (2008) Lean manufacturing performance in China: assessment of 65 manufacturing plants. *Journal of Manufacturing Technology Management*, 19(2), 217–234.

Whitworth, T. (2010) 'Transferring the success of the lean theory: quantifying the relationship between leanness and productivity in the UK construction industry', MSc dissertation, London South Bank University.

Zikmund, W. (1997) *Exploring Marketing Research*. Sixth edition. Dryden Press.

9 *Structuring and writing the dissertation*

This chapter will explain the general format for writing, organising and presenting your dissertation. These formats will provide you with a guide to structure your dissertation which should make it easier for the reader to understand what your dissertation is all about. Specific requirements for presenting the dissertation may vary from one discipline to another and from one university to another; for example, the number of copies required, format of the front cover, size of paper, typesetting and the like. However, the general formats of presentation are much the same in most disciplines, and so the main task is to make sure that you write and organise your dissertation contents correctly.

This chapter will give you guidance on how to structure and write your dissertation. It gives examples of writing an abstract, an introduction, a piece of literature review, presenting the research design and presenting the chapter of findings and conclusions. The examples given in this chapter should be treated as guidance which can serve as a model only. The contents of Chapter 9 are shown in Figure 9.1.

Typical dissertation structure

The structure of your dissertation may take the following order:

1 A page showing the title, your name, department and a copyright statement
2 Summary of figures (if any)
3 Summary of tables (if any)
4 Acknowledgements
5 Abstract
6 Introduction to the research: one chapter
7 Literature review: usually two or three chapters reviewing previous work (theory/ies and/or previous evidence)
8 Questionnaire design and method of analysis: one chapter. If the dissertation is purely based on analysing archival data, then you may name the chapter 'Procedure of data gathering'

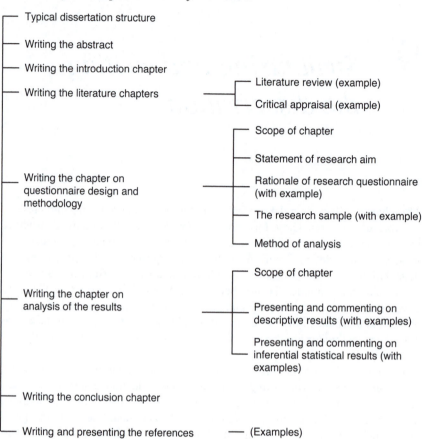

Typical dissertation structure

Writing the abstract

Writing the introduction chapter

Writing the literature chapters
— Literature review (example)
— Critical appraisal (example)

Writing the chapter on questionnaire design and methodology
— Scope of chapter
— Statement of research aim
— Rationale of research questionnaire (with example)
— The research sample (with example)
— Method of analysis

Writing the chapter on analysis of the results
— Scope of chapter
— Presenting and commenting on descriptive results (with examples)
— Presenting and commenting on inferential statistical results (with examples)

Writing the conclusion chapter

Writing and presenting the references — (Examples)

Figure 9.1 *Contents of Chapter 9.*

9 Analysis of the results: one chapter. If the dissertation is based on appraising previous work, then you may name it 'Analysis of secondary data' or 'Critical appraisal of previous work'
10 Conclusions and recommendations for further studies and practice
11 References
12 Appendices

Writing the abstract

The abstract is a brief summary of the research, usually about 200 words in length. It should give information on the research problem that was studied, the method used to study the problem (including information on the type of sample), the results, and major conclusions. The abstract should provide enough information to the examiners about your research as well as information to other readers so that they may decide whether to read the entire dissertation. The abstract should also make the dissertation easier to comprehend when it is read. Although the abstract appears at the beginning of your dissertation, you will probably want to wait until the body of the dissertation is complete before you write the abstract.

You may need several attempts before you achieve a sufficient brief. The following example fulfils all the requirements of an abstract, and might serve as a model.

Abstract (example of writing-up style)

This dissertation is about evaluating the perception of head office personnel and site managers into the factors that influence productivity on site. A critical review of the literature is structured under three chapters: (1) management; (2) motivation; and (3) experience and training. Twenty-nine factors were extracted from the above chapters headings and were assessed by 19 head office personnel and 17 site managers who were interviewed throughout the research. The survey indicated that both samples regard 'ineffective project planning' and 'constraints on a worker's performance' as the most critical factors influencing productivity. Another highly ranked factor by both samples is 'lack of integration of project information'. Given the large number of computer systems available, this must be disheartening and reflects similar findings of recent research in the use and application of IT systems.

Writing the introduction chapter

This chapter introduces the reader to the area being investigated. It basically includes most of your proposal contents. After reading the introduction, the reader should know why you decided to do the research and how you decided to go about it. In general, the introduction chapter may be composed of four sections:

1 *Rationale.* The first section of your introduction chapter starts with a description of past research which is relevant to the problem. This section may be entitled 'Nature of the problem', 'Scope of the research', 'Rationale for the research', 'Background to the problem' or the like. Here, an exhaustive review of past research is not necessary; rather you want to describe only the research and/or theoretical issues that are clearly related to your study. You should state explicitly how this previous work is logically connected to your problem. This tells the reader why your research was conducted. (See examples of rationales in Appendix 1.)

2 *Research goals.* The second section of the introduction tells the reader what your aim is, what objectives are to be achieved and what hypothesis (or key questions) is (or are) being examined. (See examples of research goals in Appendix 1.)

3 *Outline methodology and the research road map.* The third section should describe the method you used to achieve your aim and objectives. (See examples in Appendix 1.) It should also include the methodology road map. Figure 9.2 shows an example of a typical methodology road map, which is related to Proposal 2 in Appendix 1. See also Figure 2.3 as another example.

Figure 9.2 *Example of a typical road map.*

4 *Dissertation structure.* The final part of the introduction provides the reader with a short summary about the content of each chapter of your dissertation (one or two short paragraphs for each chapter).

Writing the literature chapters

The literature review is usually spread over two or three chapters. These chapters review what has been written on your topic (see Chapter 3). Haywood and Wragg (1982, p. 1) emphasised that a critical review should show that 'the writer has studied existing work in the field with insight'. The main point is that a review should provide the reader with a picture of the state of knowledge and of the main questions in the subject area being investigated.

When writing the literature review chapters ensure that you cover the following 12 points:

1   A clear title for each chapter.
2   Division of chapter into a number of sections: it starts with 'Scope of chapter' and ends with 'Critical appraisal'. (See example below and another one in Chapter 3, pp. 28–39.)
3   Sifting of information. This means that you should include only materials which are directly related to the study.
4   Clarity in writing. Be precise and clear in presenting other people's work.
5   Clearly appraising the common issues raised by previous writers in the field, as well as the similarities and differences among them.
6   Coherence in writing: the writing of the literature and indeed the whole dissertation is coherent. The material is presented in an orderly, logical progression to facilitate understanding and good reading.
7   That the grammar, punctuation and length are correct.
8   Where relevant, the use of accurate linking phrases such as 'in contrast', 'it has been reported by', 'according to', 'there is much debate about', 'another school of thought suggests', 'all evidence points towards', 'conflict in opinion was revealed when', 'two sources, namely and . . . and . . . admitted that'.
9   The inclusion of a diagram, such as Figure 3.2, or other exhibits and illustrations such as tables, charts and conceptual frameworks, that were developed by previous writers in order to clarify the point to be made as well as to make the reading more interesting.
10   Acknowledgement of the work of others. Most of the information provided in the literature chapters should be drawn from previous work. Therefore almost every statement you make in the literature review should be referenced. If you use a passage drawn from an article or book, make sure that the passage is presented as a direct quotation. There is nothing wrong with quoting another author as long as you acknowledge your source (see Referencing on pp. 158–163).
11   A good balance of old and new references.
12   A good balance of sources. For example, include material published by refereed journals, conference proceedings, reports, secondary sources and a few web sites.

Literature review (example of writing-up style)

In Chapter 3, pp. 28–39, there is an example of how to structure a typical literature chapter, but the following section will also serve as a model to show sifting, clarity and correct acknowledgement.

This section of the literature review is extracted from a study by Naoum (1989) titled 'An investigation into the performance of management and traditional form of contracts'. Proposal 2 in Appendix 1 and the methodology road map shown in Figure 9.2 are related to Naoum's study. Part of his investigation was to review previous models of the building process in order to help him develop one of his own. So Chapter 3 of Naoum's research was titled 'Review of previous models of the building process'. You may not be familiar with the field of study, and the study itself was conducted back in the 1980s, but the idea is to show you how to review previous work and what is expected from you.

Chapter 3 – Review of previous models of the building process

3.1 Scope of chapter

This chapter starts by providing a historical background to previous models of the building process and compares the ones that dealt with integration and the system theory. The model by Sidwell is discussed in more details as it will serve as a pilot for developing the author's own 'building process model'.

The chapter then discusses those characteristics of the client and the project that may affect the choice of procurement method and subsequently project performance. Case studies of previous researchers in this field are also presented in the last section of this chapter.

3.2 Historical background to previous building process models

Since the 1960s various models have been developed to investigate the effectiveness of the building team or the operation of the building process. Some researchers developed their model to show the structure of the industry such as the Tavistock model, but others were interested in showing the processes and participants involved in project development and have a temporal aspect. In other words, they show sequences of events and not instants in time. However, although the Tavistock report produced a sequential type of model, it did open the building industry's eyes up to a system approach. According to Cleland and King (1968), the system approach illustrates the interaction and interdependence between the identified variables, suggesting that an action of one variable can cause reaction on the part of others.

Among the most relevant models for this research that followed the Tavistock report are those of Morris (1972), Walker (1982), Ireland (1983), Sidwell (1982), Nahaphiet (1985), Wearne (1984), Rowlinson (1988) and Newcombe (1988).

Morris (1972) took a system view of the building industry and studied the interfaces between the design and production. He used the Tavistock report and the work of Miller and Rice on organisational boundary definition (1967) and Lawrance and Lorsch's studies of differentiation and integration (1967) as a mainspring of his research model. Morris broke down the building process into three main subprocesses which may occur sequentially or concurrently i.e. outline design, detailed design and construction. The concurrence of the building process is an indicator of the degree of integration of the building process. This integration may be modified by the managerial actions which determine the make up of the building team and the parameters by which they are guided. This managerial action may in turn be modified by the environment, which constitutes all the factors which influence the client, the building team and the building process. This provides one of the first pieces of work which approaches the problem in terms of the process as a whole and attempts to provide a rationale for actions.

Here, Morris's diagrammatical model was inserted.

Walker (1980) also adopted a system viewpoint and defined a model which is client oriented and is common to all projects. He used the technique of linear responsibility analysis to investigate decision making and appropriate organisation structures for construction project management. The model is in terms of three stages: project conception, project inception and project realisation. In recognising the non-sequential nature of the construction process, the decision points within the system adds tasks discontinuity to Miller's work (1956) on technology, territory and time.

Here, Walker's diagrammatical model was inserted

Ireland (1983) adopted Kast and Rosenweig's model (1973) of the organisation and indicated that he had reversed their proposition of management and structure being dependent systems. Ireland conducted his research on the basis that 'Technology used, structure chosen, the psychosocial aspects and the way the project is managed, will all have an effect on the achievement of goals and values subsystems'. Ireland maps these sub-systems to form a strategic control of the building process but omits discussion of who should exercise this control. It also appears that the concept of socio-technical analysis is not fully supported from his research. This is so due to the cross-sectional approach to the research method evidence for impact of the social system and the adaptive controls would be very difficult to find.

Here, Ireland's diagrammatical model was inserted.

The various models of previous researchers were studied by Sidwell (1982) who criticised them however for they infer a sequential process and do not illustrate the interactive and cyclic nature of the building process. He, therefore, identified and studied the interrelationship between 19 variables and discussed them under six main headings. These are: 1) client characteristics, 2) project characteristics, 3) project procedure, 4) building team, 5) environment 6) project success. Sidwell applied the model over 32 case studies to examine, on the one hand, the relationship between the variables: client, project building team and project procedure, which together define the organisational form. And on the other hand, variables of the organisational form are examined with variables of project success in respect to time and cost.

Here, Sidwell's diagrammatical model was inserted.

Naoum went on and stated that, Sidwell's model (1982) did not include designer characteristics nor client and contractor criteria, which are modified by the foregoing, in order to gauge performance. These criteria have been assumed previously and deemed to be project characteristics. Having said that, the success measures that Sidwell used were both subjective and objective which helps counter criticism on criteria.

Here, Naoum's diagrammatical model was inserted as shown in Figure 9.3 below.

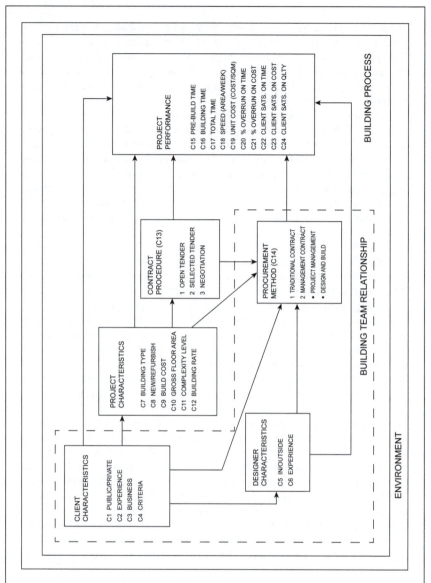

Figure 9.3   *The building process model.*

3.3. The influence of client characteristics on selecting procurement methods

Here, Naoum inserted the relevant research available that investigated the relationship between client characteristics and procurement methods such as the type of clients and criteria of project success.

3.4. The influence of project characteristics on selecting procurement methods

Here, Naoum inserted the relevant research available that investigated the relationship between project characteristics and procurement methods such as the type of projects and complexity.

3.5. Previous case studies into the performance of various procurement methods

Here, Naoum inserted the relevant case studies available that linked clients, projects, procurement methods and project performances.

3.6 Critical appraisal

Here, Naoum inserted an 'appraisal' section (approximately 500 words) to discuss the implications of the information provided in Chapter 3 on his investigation.

Note to students: The critical appraisal section is inserted at the end of every literature chapter. It can also be named 'End of chapter discussion', 'Concluding remarks' or the like. In this section, you are expected to discuss or criticise other's work using your own words. The following appraisal section is taken from a dissertation by Stuart Green (1996, pp. 34–36) on health and safety in construction. Naturally, the figures presented in the following example are outdated but the idea is to show you how to write a typical end of chapter appraisal.

Example of writing up 'end of chapter critical appraisal' section

This chapter set out to establish whether the construction industry's safety record is poor when compared to other major UK industries. A further objective of the chapter was to analyse the accidents rates and try to offer an explanation as to why these accidents occur. The first part of the chapter looked at the history of construction site accidents and showed that employment was falling (20% on the 1981 figure) and so was the incidents of accidents. Self-employment has risen by 45% over the last ten years and this has also seen a decline in the accident rate. Self-employment continues to be a grey area with regards to health and safety, but overall the combined (employed and self-employed) fatalities fell by 16% to 4.7 per 100,000 workers.

The chapter then went on to look at how at the construction industry compared with other industries with regards to health and safety. The section described how the reporting of accidents will rise with the introduction of new reporting measures but the trend will continue downwards.

Accidents rates for all industries have fallen by 25% since 1993/94, due mainly to the increase in employment in the safer industries. The construction industry saw a 20% fall in fatal injuries from 1993/94, due to the introduction of the first CDM regulations in 1994, with energy and manufacturing showing a 51% and 29% reduction respectively. The difference in accident rates between construction and manufacturing may attribute to four points as follows:

1   Factories are controlled environments
2   There is little change in manufacturing procedures or equipment
3   The manufacturing labour force remains constant
4   Hazards in factories can be remedied easier and with little cost

Accidents on construction sites usually cause multiple fatalities and injuries, such as the Ashford Disaster in the summer of 1995 when a three story building collapsed during refurbishment works killing four site workers (Construction News: 25,4,96). Accidents in factories rarely involve more than one person.

The final section of this chapter looked at accident trend in the construction industry. The figures showed that fatal and major injuries were mainly caused by fall from a height. Accident rates continue to fall but fatalities for falls remain constant. The most hazardous occupations continue to be roofing and labouring, probably due to the large amount of untrained labour employed in these sectors.

In conclusion, contents of this chapter confirm that the construction industry is still risky as far as health and safety is concerned. However, the trend for accidents is downwards and the implementation of new safety legislation such as CDM, and the increasing awareness of management, is likely to improve safety although there may be a financial cost associated with the improvement.

The following chapter explains the cost implications as a result of improving safety in the construction industry.

Writing the chapter on questionnaire design and methodology

This chapter needs to be inserted after the literature chapters. It may also be entitled 'Procedure of data gathering', 'Research design and methodology' or the like. In this chapter, you need to explain how the problem was investigated and describe the tool that you used to make the investigation (i.e. your questionnaire or the data collection format). You also need to describe the characteristics of your research sample and method of analysis. I suggest that this chapter may include the following sections.

Section 1: scope of chapter

This should be a brief explanation of what the reader will expect to read in this chapter (one or two paragraphs).

Section 2: statement of research aim

This should be a repeat of your stated aim to remind the reader what you intend to investigate (see examples of aims in Chapter 2 and in Appendix 1).

Section 3: rationale of the research questionnaire

In this section you need to rationalise your questionnaire by stating why you have asked the questions you did. Remember, your questionnaire has, say, three to five section headings and each heading contains a number of questions which are related to your research objectives. Your task, therefore, is to refer to the questionnaire, which is usually inserted in the Appendix, and discuss each section individually. For instance, what did you intend to obtain from the respondent? Which objective would you achieve by asking that group of questions? Has there been a similar type of question asked by fellow researchers? If so, refer briefly to their questionnaire or to their work. For example, in the study related to Appendix 1 on total quality management, one of the sections was entitled 'Key components of service quality'. The following rationale is taken from a dissertation by Hania Cooper, which might serve as a model (Cooper, 1995, pp. 89–91).

Questionnaire rationale: key components of service quality (example of writing up a rationale)

This section of the questionnaire lists and defines the functions of fifteen 'key components' of quality. The fifteen components comprise an adaptation of those proposed by Garvin (1987), Haywood-Farmer (1987) and Wilson (1994), amended by the author in 2010 to suit the context of a multi-disciplinary professional service firm in the construction industry.

Previous chapters have suggested that a standard accredited quality assurance (QA) system such as ISO 9001 may not sufficiently address all the pertinent aspects of quality within a professional service and it has been proposed that a market-focused approach to quality would best satisfy client requirements (Barrett 1992). It is submitted that such an approach might commence by isolating the 'key components' of service quality, such as 'competence of personnel' and 'reliability of service'. It would then be possible to establish the relative importance of such key components to the client and then use performance data to determine how far service performance matches clients expressed needs (Wilson 1994).

The company surveyed did not extend QA to marketing functions as such and, in view of the understandable importance to the firm of confidentiality in this area, detailed marketing data was excluded from the questionnaire (note that, in this particular dissertation, the student used her own firm to investigate the issues of her research). Instead, it was felt useful to use the concept of 'key components' of quality to address the respondent's own perception. Following an informal pilot survey of three construction professionals, it became clear that respondents were likely to find it too difficult and time-consuming to rate or grade each of the fifteen 'key components'. Therefore, the question was changed slightly by asking the respondents to indicate the five most important and five least important 'key components'. List of the fifteen key components and their definitions are given below:

1   Performance – defined as the provision of the basic service such as project management or quality surveying.

2   Feature – defined as supplementing basic service such as building surveying supplementing project management.

3   Reliability – defined as consistency of performance, dependability and low risk of errors.

4   Responsiveness – defined as willingness to personnel to provide service such as giving prompt service.

5   Competence – defined as profession of required skills.

6   Conformance – defined as the extent to which service meets any established standard such as Housing Corporation Scheme Development Standard.

7   Access – defined as the approachability and ease of contact.

8   Currency – defined as the ability to keep relevance and up-to-date such as with new legislation, methods and products.

9   Courtesy – defined as politeness, respect, consideration and friendliness of contact personnel.

10   Communication – defined as keeping informed in language they can understand such as explaining reasons for delays or trade-offs between service and cost.

11   Perceived quality – defined as trustworthiness, believability such as reputation of the firm or personal characteristics of contact personnel.

12   Security – defined as freedom from danger, risk or doubt such as financial security and confidentiality.

13   Understanding – defined as knowing the customers; making the effort to understand the client's needs such as specific requirements and individual attention.

14   Tangibility – defined as the physical evidence of the service such as physical facilities and equipment.

15   Costing – defined as clear pricing or accurate estimating such as known financial commitment, no hidden extras.

Notes to students

- If your research involves a theoretical framework, you need to give details of the variables or factors that you have studied. If you have designed a model, you need to give details of its components and state your argument as to how these components are interrelated. In other words, you should define the variables one by one and describe the method which you used to measure the variables [see Figure 9.3 as an example of a conceptual model designed by Naoum (1989)]. This model is related to Proposal 2 in Appendix 1.

- If your investigation is based purely on archival data and not a questionnaire, then you need to discuss the format that you used to gather the information. Remember, the archival information can be either statistical or descriptive.

Table 9.1 *Research sample: number and rate of response by category (example of writing-up style)*

Category	Questionnaires issued	Responses	% response
Directors	12 (14)	7 (14.5)	58
Associates	12 (14)	8 (17.0)	67
Constructional professionals	55 (63)	26 (54.0)	47
Admin.	8 (9)	7 (14.5)	88
Total	87	48	55

Note: Figures in brackets indicate the corresponding percentage relative to total questionnaire issued (87 = 100%), or relative to total response (48 = 100%), as applicable to that column.

Section 4: the research sample

In this section of the chapter you need to discuss the following:

1 The list that you drew your sample from.
2 The method that you used to select your sample and why.
3 If you used a survey questionnaire, state how many were sent out and how many were completed (i.e. response rate).
4 Describe the characteristics of your response sample. This can be discussed from the information gathered by the 'general' section of your questionnaire. Tables 9.1 and 9.2 show two typical examples. This part of the questionnaire was designed to establish the range of respondents in terms of annual turnover and to gain an insight into the role marketing plays within their business strategy.

Example of writing up a research sample section

The following example might serve as a model to show the style of presenting a research sample. In this example, the material is extracted from Chapter 4 of an MSc dissertation by Zoë Elizabeth Mulholland (2010). The title of this dissertation is 'An examination of sustainable construction in the recession'. Zoë wrote:

> The aim of the research sample was to cover as broad a range of perspectives as possible. The interviewees were selected from each stage of the project to include: client, architect, cost consultant and main contractor to attempt to capture these differing viewpoints. In addition, there was variation within each type of respondent group for small, medium or large company and mixture of public and private work, as well as refurbishment and new build. It is worth noting that none of the respondents were solely involved in specialist fields of work and all had a range of projects. The breakdown of respondents is set out in Table 9.2.

Table 9.2   *Overview of respondents' organisations*

Respondent	Turnover (£)	No. of staff	Sectors	Types of project	Value of projects (£)	Location
Client A	N/A (portfolio value £5.1 billion)	240	Retail park; regional shopping centres; commercial offices	Refurb; conversion; new-build	<1m, 20%; 1–10m, 20%; 10–50m, 25%; >50m, 35%	UK nationwide; France
Client B	N/A	35	Education; science research; offices; residential	Refurb; fit-out; new-build	<1m, 35%; 1–10m, 35%; 10–50m, 25%; >50m, 5%	London; Berkshire; Kent
Client C	N/A	17	Residential; 'build to let'; commercial office	Refurb; new-build	<1m, 20%; 1–10m, 70%; 10–50m, 10%; >50m, 0%	London and SE England
Architect A	N/A	34	HEI; commercial; conservation; residential – top end and social	Fit-out; refurb; new-build specialist in historical contexts	<1m, 20%; 1–10m, 60%; 10–50m, 15%; >50m, 5%	London; Oxford
Architect B	N/A	250	Science labs; health care; education – schools, HE, FE; commercial office; urban design; regeneration; interior design	Refurb; conversion; new-build	<1m, 10%; 1–10m, 20%; 10–50m, 60%; >50m, 10%	London; Manchester; Glasgow
Architect C	N/A	70	Education – school, FE, HE; health care; research; social housing	Refurb; conversion; new-build	<1m, 20%; 1–10m, 20%; 10–50m, 25%; >50m, 35%	London; Manchester; Glasgow; Belfast
Cost Manager A	N/A	2000	All	All	<1m, 10%; 1–10m, 30%; 10–50m, 30%; >50m, 30%	UK nationwide (also worldwide but not covered in interview)

Cost Manager B	TBC	100	HE; retail; commercial; health	Refurb; conversion; new-build	<1m, 30%; 1–10m, 35%; 10–50m, 35%; >50m, 0%	UK nationwide
Contractor A	N/A	45	Commercial fit-out; high-end residential; data centres; heritage/ churches; not for profit	Refurb; fit out	<1m, 55%; 1–10m, 40%; 10–50m, 5%; >50m, 0%	London
Contractor B	N/A	100	Education; commercial	Fit out; refurb	<1m, 65%; 1–10m, 30%; 10–50m, 5%; >50m, 0%	London

After showing the overall characteristics of the research sample, it is necessary to provide a short summary of all the organisations that you interviewed. In this research, there were three clients, three architects, two cost managers and two contractors.

The following extract is an example of providing some details of a respondent (Mulholland, 2010).

Client A

Client A is one of the top five commercial developers. It might have been expected that this client would only be interested in the façade of being green. However the company had a sustainability ethos engrained throughout the organisation from the top management down. Client A was one of the most enthusiastically positive respondents who saw the potential rather than the barriers to sustainable construction. The firm has an in-house sustainability department with specialist expertise but ensures that all sectors within the company have a thorough grounding in sustainable development principles so that the whole culture of the organisation embraces sustainability. As a result, Client A took the continuation of sustainable construction through the recession.

Section 5: method of analysis

This section of the research design chapter should explain how the data was analysed. If you selected the interview technique, have you used the trend approach in analysing the information or percentages? If you selected the postal survey, have you used the descriptive method of analysis or the statistical test(s)?

Writing the chapter on analysis of the results

This chapter is the core part of your dissertation and will consist of the research findings expressed by texts, figures, tables, charts, graphs and the like. It is absolutely essential to present your results clearly. I suggest the following structure for this chapter.

Section 1: scope of chapter

This section should be a brief description of what is included in the chapter.

Note to students: Chapter 8 in this book described the methods for analysing the results. If you decided to apply the descriptive method follow Section 2, part 1, below; if you decided to apply the statistical test, then follow Section 2, part 2, below; if you decided to apply both methods, then follow parts 1 and 2 below.

Section 2: analysis of the results, part 1 (the descriptive method)

This part of the dissertation will consist of questions, answers, tables, figures or charts, and comments. When writing the results section, it is best to refer back to your questionnaire. The order in which your results are presented should correspond to the order of your questionnaire. In general, the analysis of the results for the descriptive method can be presented following the format below:

1 *The question.* Here, you state the question as asked in the questionnaire.
2 *The results/finding.* Here, you present the analysis of the results in the form of table, bar chart, pie chart or a graph.
3 *Comments/interpretation.* After analysing the question and presenting the results in a table, chart or other form, you need to go beyond this step and interpret the results of your study. For instance, what do they mean to you? Are your results similar or dissimilar to the results of previous studies? If your results were different, why were they different? Did you use different subjects or use different techniques?

Below are three examples showing typical presentations of descriptive types of results. The first example (adapted from Cooper, 1995) displays results of an investigation based purely on a postal survey, the second example (adapted from Green, 1996) shows a postal survey supplemented by interviews and the third example (adapted from Naoum and Langford, 1987) is based purely on interviews.

Presenting a postal survey (example of writing-up style)

Question:
This question is related to the adequacy of the 'current' quality assurance (QA) procedures to satisfy clients' requirements and expectations. Here, the respondents were given a number of factors which can contribute to the quality of service to satisfy clients' requirements. They were asked to mark each factor with a figure 3, 2 or 1. Mark 1 means that the 'current' QA meets the client satisfaction to this particular factor. Mark 2 means that it moderately meets client satisfaction and mark 3 means it does not meet the client satisfaction at all.

Results:
The table below shows the average rate of response to the above question.

Table of results: adequacy of QA procedures to satisfy clients' requirements and expectation

		Key factors adequacy ratings (%)		
		1	*2*	*3*
Overall response				
1	Performance	84	7	9
2	Features	53	20	27
3	Reliability	59	26	15
4	Responsiveness	9	36	55
5	Competence	21	44	34
6	Conformance	43	33	24
7	Access	7	14	79
8	Currency	18	36	46
9	Courtesy	7	14	79
10	Communication	12	38	50
11	Perceived quality	0	39	61
12	Security	17	39	64
13	Understanding	17	51	32
14	Tangibles	26	35	39
15	Cost	30	45	25
Average ratings		27	32	41

Comments:

From analysis of the results shown in the above table, the following picture emerges:

1   Taking an average of the ratings over all 15 'key factors' of quality, it appears that an average of only 27 per cent of responses ranked the 'current' QA procedures as completely adequate to ensure that the clients' requirements and expectations are fully satisfied. Thirty-two per cent of the responses thought 'moderately' and 41 per cent thought that 'current' QA procedures do not cover the particular 'key factors' that were listed.

2   However, these somewhat negative results (relative to what might have been expected within a firm operating an accredited QA system) may be at least partially explained by reference to the hypothesis put forward earlier in this dissertation: 'a standard accredited QA system such as ISO 9001 may not sufficiently address all the pertinent aspects of quality'.

3   Going back to the above table, 84 per cent of respondents ranked 'performance' (that is, ensuring that the required basic service is actually performed) as fully satisfying the clients' requirements with the 'current' QA procedures.

4   Reliability was expected to be well within the remit of QA. Here, the results are a little lower: an average of 59 per cent of respondents ranked this item as fully satisfying clients' requirements, 26 per cent ranked it as moderately and 15 per cent as not at all. Further analysis of the results, into categories of responses, discloses that the majority of the low ranking came from the construction professionals which, presumably, are either genuinely critical to QA procedures or otherwise may lack knowledge as to the purposes and scope of the procedures in operation.

5   In a similar vein, the remainder of the overall 'top six' quality components appear to illustrate aspects of quality which are, indeed, less well covered by standard QA systems, such as ISO 9001. The extreme example of this is 'perceived quality', which refers to the trustworthiness of the firm or contact personnel to the client.

6   Though proposed by the majority of respondents as an important aspect of quality in the selection, retention and recommendation of the professional firm's services, not one respondent suggested that 'current' QA procedures would ensure that clients' reasonable requirements and expectations are fully satisfied in this respect. Indeed, 61 per cent indicated that they believed that 'current' QA procedures did not cover this factor. However, this finding should be treated with caution. The answers are the respondents' own perceptions and not necessarily the organisation's. A larger sample needs to be surveyed in order to confirm this finding.

7   Similar results apply to 'communication' and 'responsiveness', where 50 per cent and 55 per cent of respondents, respectively, indicated that QA procedures did not cover these key factors.

8   The respondents were also asked to rank the 'five most important' factors of quality and the 'five least important' factors that the QA procedure should take into consideration. The following were the results:

Most important factors	Least important factors
1. Reliability	1. Tangibles
2. Understanding	2. Features
3. Perceived Quality	3. Security
4. Performance	4. Currency
5. Communication	5. Conformance

Presenting postal survey supplemented by interviews (example of writing-up style)

This example is related to health and safety in construction. Postal and interview questionnaires were designed. The postal questionnaires were sent to four companies: three contractors and one construction consultancy. The recipients were mainly quantity surveyors and project managers. A total of 130 questionnaires were distributed, of which 77 completed forms were returned (60 per cent response). The returned responses were from 25 managers, 25 supervisors, 21 operatives and six consultants. All the returned questionnaires were usable. This high response to the survey was because the author had a good contact base which was formed during the professional placement. To support the findings, the student also decided to undertake interviews with the companies that responded to the survey. The following section is an extract from the analysis of the results.

Question:
This question was related to health and safety as opposed to programme time. The respondents were, therefore, asked the following question:
Do programme times imposed through contract clauses directly affect safety?
The table below presents the results.

Table of results: safety culture and programme time

	Managers		Supervisors		Operatives	
Question	Agree	Disagree	Agree	Disagree	Agree	Disagree
Do programme times imposed through contract clauses directly affect safety?	6 (65%)	9 (35%)	7 (28%)	18 (72%)	17 (80%)	4 (20%)

Comments:
The above table shows an interesting finding. It shows that, although senior managers and operatives agreed with the question, supervisors expressed a different view. Analysis of the results indicates that 65 per cent of senior site managers agreed that programme time imposed through contract clauses directly affect safety. It was commented that penalty clauses are too high and programme times are too tight, imposing a false induced money–consciousness in the industry. One manger stated during the interview:

> There is a lot of pressure brought about at the present time, clients want the shortest programme, the highest quality and lowest price. Therefore, there is an awful amount of pressure on everyone involved with the contract at site level, particularly the site managers. I agree programme times do have an effect on safety, its not a perfect world as we also put pressure on sub-contractors to get the work done, forcing them to carry out work in a dangerous manner.

When supervisors were asked the same question, 72 per cent disagreed with the question. During an interview with a supervisor, he stated:

> You can still produce to the required level and effectively if you plan safely into your production process. People tend to work better in a safer environment. Today we think more consciously about safety, so whilst there is a lot of pressure on the main contractor, the emphasis is on building it on time, with quality, within budget and in the safest manner.

Another interviewee commented:

> Under current regulations and working practices, safety is a fatal element in any construction sequence, along with staffing, materials and plant. It can not be differentiated or taken aside from. On that basis you can not regulate it, in many ways it should be in the forefront.

A third interviewee put the view that:

> You have to do it the right way, even though it will cost more or take longer. This industry is very dangerous, a serious accident will cost the contractor more than it would have cost to do it safely in the first place. The trouble is that people do not see risks until it's too late.

From the above analysis one can conclude that present contractual arrangements allow the pursuit of safety to come into conflict with the demand for the cheapest and speediest completion of a contract. The widespread use of contract penalty clauses and unrealistic productivity targets can result in a poor safety culture as it can place supervisors under considerable pressure to take the quickest and cheapest option. However, the Health and Safety issue should be part of the contractual package and, as one interviewee stated, it should be in the forefront.

Presenting results based purely on interviews (example of writing-up style)

The table in the following extract shows the results of an interview with 10 clients who were asked questions that sought to compare management contracting (MC) with the traditional method (TR) (see Appendix 6 for another example of presenting interview results in a tabulated format). Structured interviews were used to supplement data collected by questionnaire. The questionnaire was divided into seven section headings to correspond with the research objectives. The following questions were investigated:

1   Who are the clients that used MC?
2   How do client organisations view MC?
3   Why have clients used MC?
4   What are the clients' criteria of satisfaction?
5   What is the level of client satisfaction with MC?
6   Is MC favourable to traditional contracting?
7   What are the clients' attitude towards the use of MC in the future?

In this example, the questionnaire was sent to 10 client organisations prior to the interview. The organisations were coded as client A, B, C, D, E, F, G, H, I, J. Interviews were carried out by running through the questionnaire to comment on the answers of each section heading, and were documented using a mini tape-recorder. The following paragraphs provide you with a sample of a discussion that was made on the results related to question 6 above. This should give you some idea of how to write and discuss the interview results.

Table of results: responses to questions on MC versus traditional method

Response out of 10

	Yes	Same	No
1. Is MC more risky to clients?	6	2	2
2. Is MC more profitable to the contractor?	10	–	–
3. Does MC involve fewer claims?	3	4	3
4. Is MC more flexible to variations?	10	–	–
5. Does MC allow an earlier start on site?	10	–	–
6. Is MC quicker to design and build the project?	10	–	–
7. Is MC more reliable in predicting the build time?	9	1	–

8. Is MC more reliable in estimating the project cost?	6	3	1
9. Is MC cheaper?	2	4	4
10. Does MC provide more control for sub-contractors?	9	1	0
11. Does MC exercise more control over construction operations?	9	1	–
12. Does MC provide a better building design?	1	1	8

Comments:

1   As can be seen from the above table, there is a conflict of opinion concerning the risk to be absorbed by clients when dealing with a management contractor. Clients A, B and D saw the principal risk arising from the absence of a tendered lump sum price from the main contractor prior to construction. Client F claimed that:

> Clients are subject to a greater risk in respect to costs because of the staggering and phasing of orders for specific work over a longer period. While in the traditional method it was the main contractor who was taking that risk by putting a lump sum bid out at the outset. With MC the contractor is likely to settle for a smaller guaranteed profit and abandon a higher potential profit through the management of implicit risks. This balance between profit and risk has implications for clients. Larger clients may be better placed to take risks and consequently have a cheaper project.

2   All the clients that were interviewed agreed that MC is flexible in that it enables variations to the original design and specifications throughout the course of construction; they added that cost can be controlled by changes in the design without affecting project performance. Client H stated: 'with the amount of changes our organisation made for the last management contract, it would have been a disaster if we had used the traditional form of contract.'

3   However, not all clients reacted positively regarding the assertion that fewer claims arose with MC. Client D, although generally satisfied with MC, was unconvinced that MCs were less claims-conscious than traditional contracts. Clients A, B, F, H and J did not experience any differences in claims between traditional contracting and MC. This was unexpected because many articles that were published by management contractors stressed that the system involves fewer claims. In an article published by the *Building Magazine*, a management contractor stated that: 'you could run a MC without a form of contract. It is a philosophy, an attitude and a contract of trust.'

4   Frequently, the time factor was seen as one of the major advantages of MC: none of the client's that were sampled commented unfavourably about MC's time performance. All clients agreed that MC reduced the pre-contract period

by overlapping the design and construction process. This enabled the project to be completed in a shorter time than for a traditional method. However, clients A, B and D expressed the view that their experience with past MCs counted for a good deal in considering the company's other needs.

5   Conflicting attitudes about the cost factor were noted. On interviewing a large public client (A), a mismatch between its expectations and the procedures of MC with its uncertain final costs, could be observed. The client stated:

> Due to the way the public sector is organised, it is naturally biased towards caution in committing tax payers' money and ensuring that their accounting officer (i.e. Chief Executive) has answers to critical questions which might be put to him by the Public Accounts Committee.

However, a second public organisation did not feel constrained in using management contracting due to public accountability because they had to change their building procedures. According to McKinney (1983), the public sector has experienced cost reimbursement contracts for many years. This particular form of contract would certainly seem to be far more in conflict with the concept of public accountability than would a 'pure' MC, simply because the contractor carries out some of the work himself with little provision for realistic and comprehensive competition. Traditionally, the public sector has taken a narrow view and awarded contracts by means of open competition on the basis of drawings and a bill of quantities.

A private banker (B) stated that:

> there is a tendency for greater involvement of the professional consultants: the architect and quantity surveyor get involved more than they should in some work which is the MC's job. This overlapping responsibility was reflected in higher fees being paid.

Four private clients had a fairly positive attitude toward the cost performance of MC. Clients C, E, F and G had a fairly positive attitude toward the cost performance of MC. One distinguishing characteristic amongst this group was that low costs were not considered as essential for client satisfaction.

6   None of the clients interviewed felt that MC produced a better building design than the traditional method, but most clients stated that they did not choose a MC for that reason in the first place.

7   Finally, the management contractors and clients who participated in the study criticised many contracting organisations for entering MC without the right personnel. Client C noted that:

> although from the client's point of view, the intention is to integrate them with the professional team of architect, structural engineers and quantity surveyors at an early stage in the proceedings to gain the advantage of their know-how within the building industry, many have not yet understood or chosen to understand this change in status and merely regard themselves as administrative middle-men in between the sub-contractors and client and

the professional team and thus do not inject any creative ideas, which is one of the objects of the exercise and is indeed the reason why certainly in our case, after a careful selection process, we bring them into the proceedings at the earliest possible stage.

Section 2: analysis of the results, part 2 (test of correlation and/ or association)

If you applied inferential statistical tests, this part of the dissertation will then consist of hypothesis testing, tables of correlation or association and interpretation of the results. The table in the following example shows an example of a survey extracted from an MSc dissertation investigating whether there are significant differences in opinions between head office personnel and site managers on factors that influence construction productivity (Hackmann, 1993). Several productivity factors were extracted from the literature review and were assessed by 19 head office personnel and 17 site managers. The findings were presented as follows.

Example 1 – Presenting results using inferential method of analysis (manual calculation)

The research question

Do site managers and the head office perceive productivity factors differently?

The research hypothesis

There are significant differences in perceptions between head office personnel and site managers with regard to factors impairing productivity. These differences are related to management techniques, resource management, motivation and experience.

The null hypothesis

There is no difference in ranking to productivity factors between head office personnel and site managers.

Statement of hypothesis testing

The following table of results shows that there is a high correlation in the ranking between the two samples. Hence, the null hypothesis can be accepted concluding that head office personnel and site managers do not perceive productivity factors differently. The table also shows that there seems to be an overall agreement by both samples with regard to productivity factors (Rho=0.78). This indicates that high ranking by head office personnel to the productivity factors correspond to high ranking by site managers to the same factors, and vice versa.

Comments

Based on the above findings, the following interpretations are made:

1 The respondents identified 'ineffective project planning' as the most crucial factor likely to impair construction productivity. This finding supports Borcherding's notion in that 'the planning/design level is probably the key communication link in the hierarchy model between the "reality" of the site construction level and the "abstract" of the policy and programme levels. The planning/design level becomes the controlling element in the industry's effort to translate productivity information from above into a common language with a terminology meaningful to the desired audience' (Borcherding and Garner, 1981).

The survey results: analysis of the survey result is shown in the table below.

Productivity factors	Head office rank (A)	Site managers rank (B)	Difference in ranks $di = (A–B)$	Difference in ranks square $di^2 = (A–B)^2$
1. Head office factors				
Lack of integration of project information	5	3	2	4
Ineffective project planning	1	1	0	0
Poor scheduling of project	8	11	23	9
Under direction of employees	10	9	1	1
Exclusion of site managers from contract meetings	8	10	22	4
Poor selection of project personnel	11	12	21	1
Lack of consultation in decision making	8	13	25	25
2. Resource management effectiveness				
Difficulties with the procurement of material	5	3	2	4

Disruption of site program	5	8	23	9
Discrepancies with technical information	10	6	4	16
Ignorance/lack of knowledge of project technology	12	6	6	36
3. Motivational factors				
Low salary	13	11	2	4
Constraints on a worker's performance (work environment)	2	3	21	1
4. Experience and knowledge factors				
Lack of experience and training	3	6	23	9
Poor knowledge of scientific techniques (workers)	14	14	0	0

Total $di^2 = 123$

$$\rho = \frac{6\sum d_i^2}{N(N^2-1)} = 1 - \frac{6 \times 123^2}{15(225-1)} = 0.78$$

$P < 0.005$

Another highly scored factor within this section, was 'lack of inter-unit integration of project information', which is a factor related to the site-level construction information system. This emphasises the importance of focusing on information required to drive the building process in addition to the technical information for design-related problems.

The difference in perception between the two samples was registered in the area of 'lack of consultation in decision making'. It was identified that head office personnel assigned a moderate score to this factor while site managers gave it a low scoring.

2   The factors that seem to be of importance to both samples in questions related to resource management effectiveness are that of 'difficulties with the procurement of materials' and 'disruption of site programme'. As far as material mismanagement is concerned, comments from site managers indicated that most acute problems, caused by material mismanagement, are with material supply and storage, which had a great impact on the sequence of work, and rework due to disruptions. This finding adds further support to Thomas's studies

(Thomas *et al.*, 1989, 1992) who found that the average daily productivity for the non-disrupted days was 0.44 work hours/sqm, whereas disrupted days had an average productivity of 2.16 work hours/sqm. This finding demonstrates the average degree of productivity improvement that can be achieved through better resource management control.

With regard to 'disruption of site programmes', this factor can cause delay in executing the work and prevent optimising utilisation of available resources. Timely input from all levels of management can reduce the risk of overlooking activities necessary to complete the project. Therefore, delays contributing to lowering a worker productivity can be reduced by planning the work to efficiently utilise manpower.

There was disagreement between both samples on 'discrepancies with technical information' and 'ignorance of project technology'. Head office personnel did not regard them as highly important, while site managers did. It was noted by site managers that waiting time due to discrepancies with technical information can be reduced by providing adequate supervision at the work place.

3   In reviewing the results described by previous researchers, there would appear to be a difference in views over whether work force motivation can affect construction productivity. Several behavioural and physiological researchers indicated that the expenditure of effort by a worker is the physical manifestation of motivation; the greater a worker's motivation, the greater his/her expenditure of effort. Ranking on questions related to motivation show that there was little support to the factor of 'low salary'. However, a substantial proportion of both samples were in agreement with the statement that 'constraints on worker's performance arising from ineffective management will affect their motivation at work and consequently influences worker's productivity'. This finding is congruent with Borcherding's conclusions (Borcherding and Oglesby, 1975; Borcherding and Garner, 1981) in that the major sources of dissatisfaction commonly expressed, by both tradespeople and supervisors, are problems related to delay and reworking. According to Thomas *et al.* (1989), frequently cited problems include the lack of tools, materials, delayed decisions, late information and changes to orders. The link between satisfaction and improved productivity is based upon the impact that such conditions are assumed to have on workers' and supervisors' motivation. It can be concluded, therefore, that individual needs for opportunities for advancement as well as the satisfaction from the work itself can be frustrating and, consequently, the potential for significant productivity gains is seen by the respondents as being thwarted by inappropriate or inadequate managerial actions.

4   Results to questions related to knowledge and experience show that both samples regarded 'lack of experience and training' as highly influential to site productivity. Obviously, each task requires specific skills and knowledge of how to use these skills. This finding ties closely with earlier results of this research regarding 'ineffective planning' and 'material mismanagement'. On the other hand, both samples do not regard 'scientific knowledge by workers' as crucial.

Example 2 – Presenting results using inferential method of analysis (using the SPSS software package) (also see example 2 in Chapter 8, pp. 121–125)

This example is based on a study that was conducted at London South Bank University by Brian Hemmings in 2009, and the result was later published in 2011 (Naoum *et al.*, 2011).

Title of research

Is there a correlation between contractors' health and safety (H&S) performance and their profit margin?

Aim

To demonstrate in a graphical format, the relationship between the performance of H&S on site and the profit margin of the contractor.

Brief research methodology

To achieve this aim, data from 22 construction projects was collected, in particular: (1) data project information; (2) procurement method; (3) start and end date; (4) actual completion date; (5) contract value; (6) final account value; (7) H&S audits and scores; (8) percentage of profit.

For each of the projects, the percentage increase or decrease of its final cost against its final value was calculated so that the percentage of profit could be analysed. Health and safety audits were carried out on all projects every month by either the project manager or the surveyor of the individual project. In order to conduct the audit, each site was issued with an H&S register and within the register there were 39 different sections covering a wide range of site specific tasks, requirements and statutory duties. Pertinent to the specific site, each site was audited once a month to check whether the tasks and duties, as set out in the register, had been carried out.

The information garnered from the audit was then transferred to a spreadsheet which monitored whether the site agent had been compliant or non-compliant with each section of the register.

Measurement of health and safety score

The H&S score is, perhaps, one of the most important headings. It gives the average score throughout the duration of the project. The score is calculated out of 100 per cent, with 100 per cent being the highest score possible. If a project scored 100 per cent it could be concluded that it had performed brilliantly, throughout its duration. The H&S score was calculated by analysing the monthly audits of the H&S register; this is explained in greater detail in the following paragraphs.

The H&S register comprises 39 different sections which place a duty on the site agents to either check certain tasks have been completed or to ensure statutory

---

guidelines have been adhered to. Once a month, either the project manager or project surveyor will audit the register to check that the site agent has complied with the relevant sections pertinent to the project. The sections within the register include: (1) Site commencement; (2) Accident reporting; (3) Asbestos; (4) Cartridge tools; (5) Control of noise; (6) COSHH; (7) Demolition; (8) Electricity on site; (9) Excavation/groundwork; (10) False work; (11) Fire prevention; (12) General H&S; (13) HFL & LPG; (14) Site visits; (15) Lifting operations; (16) Manual handling; (17) Permits to work; (18) PPE; (19) Piling; (20) Construction phase plan; (21) Risk assessment; (22) Road works; (23) Scaffold/work platforms; (24) Site induction; (25) Site instructions; (26) Site security; (27) Statutory records; (28) Steel fabrication; (29) Subcontractor safety; (30) Traffic management; (31) Training/toolbox talks; (32) Under/over ground services; (33) Waste management; (34) Welfare; (35) Work equipment; (36) Working at high level; (37) Working in confined spaces; (38) Young persons; (39) Environment.

The project manager or surveyor fills out a report that highlights which sections have or have not been complied with. This information was transferred to a monthly audit summary which plots each of the sections that the project had been non-compliant with.

This summary data was then extracted to a table which scheduled out the complete duration of the project month by month. For every month an H&S score was calculated by plotting the number of non-compliant sections out of 39. The amount of compliant sections were then divided by 39 and multiplied by 100 to get a percentage out of 100.

Measurement of profit percentage

The percentage of profit made is the second most important heading as it gives the actual amount of profit the project made. This was done by calculating the difference in the actual cost against the final out-turn value (final account sum), dividing it into the cost and multiplying by 100 to get a percentage.

Presentation of results

Table 9.3 below gives a breakdown of each project's final account, its out-turn cost, its H&S score and the percentage of profit. The results show that out of the 22 projects, 16 made a profit and they each had H&S scores higher than 70 per cent, with the average score being 95 per cent and the average profit margin 20 per cent. Fourteen had an H&S score of higher than 95 per cent; all but one made a loss. The average profit was 20 per cent.

Amongst the 16 projects that had an H&S score of 90 per cent or higher, all but two projects made a profit. The average profit margin was 18 per cent.

For the six non-profit making projects, their average health and safety score was 84 per cent. Amongst them, four projects made a loss with an average H&S score of 78 per cent.

Overall, the average score was 92 per cent with the average amount of profit at 13 per cent.

Table 9.3   *Project values with Health & Safety Score and Profit Margin.*

Proj	Final Account (£)	Out turn Cost (£)	H&S Score (%)	Profit (%)
1	346,039	295,176	90	17
2	403,450	420,000	100	−4
3	554,950	423,863	99	31
4	1,250,000	1,098,166	100	14
5	628,000	628,000	100	0
6	3,250,000	3,050,000	96	7
7	4,152,000	2,875,000	98	44
8	1,148,864	1,062,446	99	8
9	260,212	243,716	99	7
10	1,675,428	1,675,428	89	0
11	190,018	152,515	99	25
12	6,885,812	5,900,000	79	17
13	2,375,012	2,300,000	96	3
14	6,000,000	3,500,000	99	71
15	2,945,431	2,471,812	96	19
16	765,057	837,842	52	−9
17	1,655,476	1,701,419	70	−3
18	449,054	445,000	81	1
19	1,675,428	1,650,428	88	2
20	2,951,619	3,179,997	91	−7
21	2,350,000	1,735,799	95	35
22	221,534	191,849	98	15

Source: reproduced from Naoum *et al*. (2011).

Calculating the strength of the relationship using the SPSS package

In order to calculate the significance of the correlation, the following steps were taken:

1   Formulate the research hypothesis: 'Projects that score high in health and safety performance will result in a higher rate of profit margin.'

2   By implication, the null hypothesis is: 'There is no significant relationship between health and safety performance and the profit margin of the contractor.'

The calculation of the correlation coefficient was performed using the SPSS package as shown in Appendix 5.

Figure 9.4 demonstrates the scatter plot of Profit on project (y) against H&S score (x). Regression analysis of profit margin on H&S score suggested that there is no significant linear relationship ($R^2 = 0.1677$, $p > 0.05$). Instead, curvilinear regression analysis in SPSS revealed that profit best correlates with H&S score with $R^2 = 0.4556$ at $P < 0.001$ in an exponential growth curve model with a plausible equation (1) of:

Figure 9.4 *Results of curvilinear regression analysis.*

$$y = e^{6.369 - \frac{320.703}{x}} - 10 \tag{1}$$

Concluding comments of this section

Although projects with a full H&S score did not all yield an overall profit, which suggests profitability depends on factors other than H&S management, projects that had an H&S sore of above 95 per cent had an average profit margin of 20 per cent. As the H&S score got lower so did the average corresponding amount of profit. It can therefore be concluded that the better the H&S score of a project the more profit that project is likely to make. It can also be said that the worse performing sites, in terms of score, actually make less profit. The results show that there is a link that can be drawn between H&S performance and profit.

The results also back up previous research and literature by the Health and Safety Executive that suggested investing in health and safety management can be a major contributor to business success.

Writing the conclusion chapter

The conclusion chapter is the end product of your investigation and should not be confused with the results chapter or a summary. It should be tied very closely with your introduction chapter. Before writing the conclusion chapter, you need to read your research aim, objectives and hypothesis (or key questions), and start to conclude what you investigated within the broader context of your proposal. Start reading the whole dissertation thoroughly and make a note of key issues or findings. The contents of the conclusion chapter should include the following:

1 Scope of chapter (one or two paragraphs).
2 Comments on the research objectives. Here take each objective in turn and conclude what you have achieved in each objective. Are your conclusions similar or dissimilar to those of previous writers in the subject area?
3 Comments on the research hypothesis or the research questions (whichever is applicable). Here state whether your investigation proved or disproved your research hypothesis.
4 Achievement of the research aim. Remember that in your proposal as well as in the introduction chapter, you provided a statement of aim which was phrased as if you were to deliver some kind of a product such as to provide professional guidelines, to develop a conceptual framework, to construct a comparative table, to design a management system, to develop a chart or to derive a mathematical formula.

   In this section of the conclusion chapter, you need to demonstrate the achievement of that stated aim. Appendix 7 shows an example of an achieved aim which is related to Proposal 2 in Appendix 1 and also to the methodology road map in Figure 9.2. The aim of this research was 'To provide a guideline to clients on the selection of the appropriate procurement method for their projects.'
5 Personal recommendations (practical) as to what should and should not be done: perhaps a modification of your conceptual model or a development of a new framework.
6 Limitations of your research. Here, state what difficulties you were faced with throughout the research process that hindered you from achieving part of your objectives.
7 Further research.

Writing the references/bibliography

There are several different ways of citing references in your dissertation and describing the sources of your references, such as the Harvard (author–date) system and the Vancouver (numerical) system. Guides can be found in most libraries. It has to be stressed that it is essential that you use references in accordance with the guidance issued by your course, which may be included in unit guides or as a separate school publication. The following is a guide to issues about referencing that often cause some puzzlement. Before describing how to compile your references, general information on using the Harvard system in your dissertation is provided below.

What does 'referencing' mean?

References to the particular source are required if you draw upon another writer's ideas in your dissertation, or if you make a direct quote. Important reasons for referencing are:

1 to acknowledge other people's ideas;
2 to show that you are not just giving your own opinions but are also including those of other people;
3 to illustrate a point or to offer support for an argument you want to make;
4 to enable readers of your work to find the source material.

A well-used quotation can make a point clearly and concisely, but try not to overuse quotations. It is important that you demonstrate your understanding of what you have read and are able to develop your own ideas by putting points or arguments into your own words.

How many references do I need to make?

There is no hard and fast rule as to how many references are required in a dissertation and much may depend upon the topic. Generally it would be impossible and unwieldy if you referenced every point you made but general guidance is that the main points or arguments you present, and especially direct quotes or ideas drawn directly from other people's work, should be acknowledged and referenced. Failure to give credit to other people's work appropriately could be considered plagiarism.

What is plagiarism?

Plagiarism is to 'use the thoughts, writings, inventions, etc. of another person as one's own' (Soanes and Stevenson, 2004). Usually we are all formulating our own ideas from different information heard and read, but plagiarism involves a deliberate attempt to pass off someone else's ideas as your own, or to copy sections or chunks of texts from another's work without attempting to put these ideas into your own words or to acknowledge the sources. It is a form of theft and is certainly regarded as a serious offence in educational settings.

How do I incorporate references and quotations into my dissertation?

Using the Harvard system you must always give the author(s) and year of publication of your source. References can be incorporated into the text in a variety of ways, such as in the following examples:

- In the following example you are making a statement in your own words and giving a reference for the source of your ideas or support for your argument:

According to Haralambos and Holborn (1990), there are variations in the way deviancy can be defined in society today.

Further examples:

A recent television programme discussed . . . (BBC, 1994)
Research undertaken by Stainton Rogers (1991) indicated that . . .
Statistics show that . . . (Health lines, 1994)

- In the following example you are making a direct quote (note that you must include the page number also):

Haralambos and Holborn state that 'the family has been seen as a universal institute, an inevitable part of human society' (Haralambos and Holborn, 1990, p. 453).

- With a longer quote it is generally preferred to indent the whole quote to make it clear:

Even though attitudes of the clients are influenced by the experiences of individual organisations, there seems to be room for improvement in the management contracting system. One such shift would be for the construction industry, and in particular the management contractors, to adopt a professional – as opposed to a commercial – role. Yet this change may be shaped by clients, who can do much to fashion events by matching their own procedures to the requirements of the procurement method they have chosen. Project performance is often elusive, but the appropriate mix of client control and procurement method can make it less so.

(Shamil Naoum, 1994, p. 704)

How do I refer to a work which I have not seen myself but which is referred to in something that I have read?

These are known as secondary or second-hand references. Ideally they should be avoided as you should have read the original items yourself but, if it is unavoidable, it is important to make clear that this is a secondary reference, as follows:

In an article of 1991 Wilford also maintains that Columbus's treatment of native people following his conquests is frequently seen in an ambiguous light (cited by Ransby, 1992).

The 'cited by' statement makes it clear that you have not seen the item by Wilford, only what Ransby says about it. Details of the item by Ransby will then appear in the reference list at the end of your dissertation as this is the source of your information, that is:

RANSBY, B. (1992) Columbus and the making of historical myth. *Race and Class* 3(3) Jan–Mar, pp. 79–86.

Wilford must not appear in your reference list as you have not seen this article.

Compiling the reference list and bibliography

What is the difference between a reference list and a bibliography?

A reference list contains details of any item you have referred to or quoted from in your dissertation. A bibliography is a list of items you have made use of in preparing your dissertation, but not referred to in your text.

How do I set out my reference list and bibliography?

Both lists are placed at the end of your dissertation and usually the reference list appears first. Both lists will be arranged in alphabetical order of author (following the Harvard system), and details given should be presented in a consistent format. Usually it is not necessary to include in your bibliography any item already listed in your reference list.

What details are required and where do I find these details?

Details required for a book can be found on the front and reverse of the title page, which is usually the first or second unnumbered page inside the book.

Details for a book should be set out in the following order: Author, Initials (year) *Title*. Edition (if later than first). Place of publication (Town): Name of publisher. Example:

NAOUM, S. (1998) *Dissertation Research & Writing for Construction Students*. Oxford: Butterworth-Heinemann.

Details required for a journal article can usually be found on the contents list, the front cover or the article itself. Details for a journal article should be set out in the following order:

Author, Initials (year) Title of article. *Name of journal.* Volume number (Issue number), Date of issue, First and last pages. Example:

NAOUM, S. (1994) Critical Analysis of Time and Cost of Management and Traditional Contracts. *Journal of Construction Engrg. and Mgnt,* 120(4), Dec. pp. 687–705.

It is not necessary to put authors' names in capitals but it can help to make them stand out. Equally it can help readers if you underline titles or use a different typeface.

How do I give details from an edited book when the chapters are by different authors?

It is important to give details for each of the chapters you have referred to or used. The details of the chapter come first and then details of the book as a whole. Example:

BREWSTER, C. (1992) Managing industrial relation in TOWERS, B. (ed.) *A Handbook of Industrial Relations Practice: Practice and law in the employment relationship.* 3rd edn. London: Kogan Page. Ch. 8.

Points to note

1 *Authors*: If there are more than two authors it is acceptable to put the first author listed followed by *et al.* (which means 'and others') in the text. If you need to refer to two or more items written by the same author in the same year use letters to differentiate the items, for example Smith (1994a), Smith (1994b).

2 *Dates*: Occasionally items do not give a date of publication, in which case you put the abbreviation n.d. in brackets (this stands for 'no date'). This shows that you have checked for the date and not just forgotten to include it.

3 *Edition*: Include edition statements only if later than first. No edition statement indicates that it is a first edition. Make sure that you match the edition statement with the correct year of publication. This should be indicated clearly on the reverse of the title page.

4 *Page numbers*: You should always put a page number for a quote. In some cases the point you make might be referred to on a specific page or between specific pages (e.g. pp. 172–175). Sometimes it may be difficult to give specific page numbers as an argument may be supported by the item as a whole.

How do I describe a government report or an Act of Parliament?

Most reports will have a government department, body or committee as an author, or may be well known by the name of the chairperson of the group or committee. With Acts of Parliament it is acceptable, and often easier, to cite the title of the Act in your text and then to include it in the reference list in alphabetical order of the first main word of the Act. Examples:

SECRETARY OF STATE FOR HEALTH (1992) Health of the nation: a strategy for health in England. London: HMSO.
EDUCATION ACT 1988. London: HMSO.

NB: HMSO is frequently the publisher of government reports and of all Acts. This abbreviation is acceptable. However, it is incorrect to describe HMSO as the author of a report, even if there is no clear author.

What about describing other types of material such as videos, leaflets and internet-based resources?

These are important sources of information but sometimes can be harder to describe. The golden rule always is to describe items as fully and clearly as possible, and in a consistent format. In the case of television/radio programmes make sure you note the date and channel of transmission. Unless self-evident it may be useful to indicate that an item is an audio- or video-cassette.

In the case of leaflets, the author is often the organisation publishing the leaflet. Example:

London South Bank University (n.d.) *Referencing using the Harvard System: frequently asked questions.* London.

Finally, remember to:

- Keep a careful note of all your sources as you prepare your dissertation.
- Make a note of book details before you return the book to the library.
- Make sure you have the details you require on any photocopies you make.
- Make sure you are referencing according to any guidelines set by your course.

This may seem like hard work but it is a vital part of your dissertation and you may lose marks for incorrect referencing.

Summary

This chapter provided the guidelines that simplify the writing and organising of the dissertation material. It illustrated the logic of structuring the dissertation. In general, a dissertation is composed of three main parts. Part I covers the introduction chapter as well as two or three chapters of literature review. Part II covers the research design. Part III covers analysis of the results and conclusions. The main points to remember are:

1 The abstract should be brief, stating what you are investigating, how, and the main finding(s).
2 The introduction chapter should state the problem, purpose of study, aim, objectives, hypothesis and contents of the dissertation.
3 The literature chapters should be divided into sections with specific themes. All quotations must be acknowledged. At the end of each chapter, you need to appraise (critically or otherwise) the material that you included.
4 The research design chapter should give the technique that you used to gather the information, the rationale to the questionnaire, the source of data, characteristics of the sample, the method of analysis and/or the format for presenting the findings.
5 The results chapter should clearly state the issues under investigation, the findings, and comments on or interpretation of the results.
6 The conclusion chapter should comment on the objectives and hypothesis/es that are stated in the introduction chapter.
7 The references/bibliography should follow a uniform system.
8 Other mechanics of presenting a dissertation, such as length and page formatting, should be followed in accordance with the rules and regulations set by your institution.

References and additional reading

American Psychological Association (1974) Publication manual. *Journal of Personality and Social Psychology*, 29, 80–85.

Bell, J. (2005) *Doing Your Research Project: A Guide for First-Time Researchers in Education and Social Science*. Fourth edition. McGraw-Hill International.

Cooper, H. (1995) 'Quality assurance in practice', BSc dissertation, School of Construction, London South Bank University.

Green, S. (1996) 'An investigation into the effect of safety culture and site operatives behaviour on construction site safety in the UK', BSc dissertation, School of Construction, London South Bank University.

Hackman, J. (1993) 'An investigation into the factors that impair the productivity of site managers', MSc Dissertation, School of Construction Economics and Management, London South Bank University.

Haywood, P. and Wragg, W. (1982) *Evaluating the Literature, Rediguide 2*. University of Nottingham, School of Education.

Hemmings, B. (2009) 'A study into the correlation between contractor's Health and Safety performance and contractors profit: Can effective safety management improve a contractor's profit margin?', MSc dissertation, Department of the Built Environment, London South Bank University.

Howard, M. (1995) 'Marketing and the quantity surveyor: Understanding clients', MSc dissertation, School of Construction, London South Bank University.

Mulholland, Z.E. (2010) 'An examination of sustainable construction in the recession', MSc dissertation, Department of the Built Environment, London South Bank University.

Naoum, S. (1989) 'An investigation into the performance of management contracts and the traditional methods of building procurement', PhD thesis, Brunel University, Middlesex.

Naoum, S. (1991) 'Procurement and project performance: A comparison of management and traditional contracting'. Occasional Paper No. 45, Chartered Institute of Building.

Naoum, S. and Hackman, J. (1996) Do site managers and the head office perceive productivity factors differently? *Journal of Engineering, Construction and Architectural Management*, 3, March/June, 147–159.

Naoum, S. and Langford, D. (1987) Management contracting: The clients' view. *Journal of Construction Engineering and Management*, 111(3), Sept, 369–384.

Naoum, S., Hemmings, B., and D. Fong (2011) 'Is there a correlation between contractor's health and safety performance and their profit margins?', 6th International Structural Engineering and Construction Conference (ISEC – 6), 21–26 June, Zurich. Paper ID S1-C32.

Soanes, C. and Stevenson, A. (2004) *Concise Oxford English Dictionary*. Oxford University Press.

South Bank University (n.d.) *Referencing Using the Harvard System: Frequently Asked Questions*. London South Bank University.

10 *Dissertation supervision and assessment*

Once you have decided on the topic of your study and your proposal gets approved, your department should then appoint a personal supervisor for you. It is therefore important to know the role of your supervisor and what is expected from him/her.

This chapter will discuss the basics of what you should expect from your supervisor. It first explains what the role of the supervisor is and what it is not. Second, it illustrates how you may plan your dissertation and finally how would you expect to be assessed in the end.

It has to be stressed, however, that the information provided in this chapter is what is known as the standard, and different institutions might have other requirements and regulations.

Getting started

Most universities run dissertation workshops that cover a range of issues such as identification of research questions, assessing whether the topic is researchable, planning and undertaking a literature review, research strategies, research techniques, data analysis, writing and structuring the dissertation.

Following these workshops, each student will then submit a dissertation proposal (similar to the ones shown in Appendix 1). This proposal usually gets approved by the dissertation tutor (a person who is responsible for the dissertation module in your department).

After that, the dissertation tutor will allocate you a supervisor to look after your work. This allocation takes place during your study term and usually in the middle of the last term.

Once you are allocated a supervisor, it is your responsibility to arrange meetings with him/her. It is advisable to arrange a meeting with your supervisor as early as possible. Your supervisor should have a copy of the approved proposal, which forms the basis of discussion in these initial meetings.

It is strongly recommended that students and supervisors should meet at least twice following their initial meetings (proposal stage): once in the middle of the process to discuss progress, and once in the final stages to discuss the final draft. Additional meetings may be required for some students to discuss progress and drafts of individual chapters as they are written (see Dissertation supervision log section on p. 170). These additional contacts may take place electronically, for example by e-mail.

Note to students: It is unlikely that you can change your allocated supervisor. On rare occasions, students may find it difficult to work with the allocated supervisor. In such cases, the dissertation tutor should act as a mediator to resolve the differences through some agreed action plan. If this fails, then a different allocation should be arranged. It must be stressed, however, that, if this unlikely situation occurs, it should be acknowledged and sorted as soon as possible before it is too late. Your supervisor is a resource, so use him/her to your advantage. He/she has normally been allocated time by the department to supervise you, so make sure you take advantage of this, but bear in mind that your supervisor is there to help you, not to do your work for you.

The role of the supervisor

The role of supervisor is to guide students towards the production of their dissertation by discussing each part of the process. The role of your supervisor can be summarised as follows:

1 To help you to develop your idea/topic further.
2 To help you to focus on your aim and objectives.
3 To help you sharpen your research questions and/or hypotheses.
4 To provide you with guidance about the appropriate research approach.
5 To approve your questionnaire before you distribute it to respondents.
6 To assist you in structuring your dissertation.
7 To discuss and monitor your progress.
8 To provide you with feedback on your chapters. This may be in the form of criticisms of your work.
9 To help you to present the final dissertation.

What is not the role of the supervisor?

From the above section, it is clear that your supervisor's duty is to guide you so that you can produce your best work. However, there are certain limitations on what is expected from your supervisor. These can be summarised as follows:

* Supervisors are not obliged to act as proofreaders of your work.
* Students should not expect their supervisor to provide detailed feedback on more than one draft of each chapter (writing a dissertation is not an iterative process), or to correct spelling, grammar, punctuation and so on.
* It is recommended that supervisors read the whole of the final draft before submission. However, if they do so, it is on the understanding that the result of the final examination is not in any way pre-judged.

- Supervisors are not to assist with continual revision until the dissertation has acquired a certain grade that you may have as a target. Therefore, the supervisor's approval of your progress cannot be taken to imply any particular grade or classification. It is not expected that you request this from your supervisor at any stage of the dissertation module.

Planning your dissertation

In order not to let things drift, it is absolutely crucial to plan and time-manage your dissertation process. Figure 10.1 is an example of a work schedule for a typical dissertation.

Notes to students

- Many of the above activities may overlap or take place before or after the suggested activities within the work schedule. For example, writing your literature chapters may take place while you analyse your questionnaire.
- There might be other activities involved in your research. For example, your dissertation might include a separate chapter on 'Discussion'. Alternatively, you might wish to include a separate chapter titled 'Critical appraisal of literature' and insert it after Chapter 3 in the suggested work schedule shown in Figure 10.1. Your dissertation topic may necessitate a further chapter of literature review, so you should allow time for it.

Therefore, you need to design your work schedule to fit your own needs.

Dissertation supervision log

As mentioned above, you should arrange 'formal' meetings with your supervisor at least three times throughout the whole process. I call them 'formal' because, at each of these meetings, it is recommended that you fill out a 'log' form like the one shown in Figure 10.2. Some institutions even require these logs to be signed by the supervisor.

The purpose of these log forms is to keep a record of your progress and to act as milestones. You can arrange as many meetings as you and your supervisor think necessary, but the three essential meetings are:

Meeting 1: Proposal stage
Meeting 2: Progress
Meeting 3: Final draft

Notes to students

- You may need more than one progress meeting.

Activity	Planned starting date	Tick when completed	Comments
1. Identify a topic			
2. Undertake background reading			
3. Identify working title			
4. Prepare dissertation proposal			
5. Proposal approved by dissertation tutor			
6. First meeting with your supervisor after proposal approved			
7. Undertake literature review			
8. Building up your literature file			
9. Designing a questionnaire (if applicable)			
10. Designing a data collection format for secondary data (if applicable)			
11. Questionnaire or data collection format approved by your supervisor			
12. Building up a list of respondents for postal survey or interviews			
13. Sending out questionnaire			
14. Conducting interviews (if applicable)			
15. Collating secondary data for analysis (if applicable)			
16. Analysing the questionnaire, interviews or secondary data			
17. Write Chapter 1 – Introduction			
18. Write Chapter 2 – Literature			
19. Write Chapter 3 – Literature			
20. Write Chapter 4 – Research design and methodology			
21. Write Chapter 5 – Findings			
22. Write Chapter 6 – Conclusions			
23. Write list of references			
24. Write abstract			
25. Give final draft to a critical reader to proofread			
26. Give final draft to your supervisor for final comments and feedback			
27. Write acknowledgement			
28. Insert appendices			
29. Insert list of tables and figures			
30. Send to binding			
31. Submit			

Figure 10.1   *Example of a typical dissertation work schedule.*

• After you complete the log form it is strongly recommended that you send a copy to your supervisor for information and filing. You can do this by electronic means.

Dissertation Supervision Log

Student's Name _____   Supervisor's Name _____

Meeting Number _____   Date:_____

Issues Discussed/Comments:

1.

2.

3.

4.

5.

Figure 10.2   *Example of a typical log form.*

Actions Required:

1.

2.

3.

4.

5.

Figure 10.2   *(Continued)*

Dissertation assessment: qualities in assessing at MSc level

In the following notes an overview is given about the qualities expected in the three marking bands (distinction, pass and fail) at London South Bank University (Buckley and Naoum, 2005). I cannot stress enough that this is only an example of assessing the quality of dissertations at MSc level and it may not be considered the norm. Other universities or courses, such as BSc, may apply different qualities of assessment.

There are three aspects to consider when assessing the qualities of a masters dissertation:

1 descriptions of qualities;
2 judgement of the degree of difficulty; and
3 key words. They are designed as prompts for the marking teams and the qualities should be considered in combination and should not be interpreted mechanically.

1. Descriptions of qualities

Distinction (70 marks or over)

The dissertation will contain some originality in the research subject chosen or in the research questions that have been developed. The research will show strong evidence in at least one of the degrees shown in aspect 2 below. The study will demonstrate a sustained and rigorous use of theoretical/conceptual or empirical evidence to support the argument or discussion. Definitions and assumptions will be clear throughout the work. There will be strong evidence of critical analysis, judgement, originality or interpretation.

There will be discussion of methods and sources that link the research design or research approach to an appropriate literature about research methods. There will be reflection about the research process or the questions for further research, which are suggested by the findings of the study. There must be an argument put forward to support the methods adopted.

The study will be well structured and written in good English. A coherent and well-considered argument will be developed. Accurate referencing of sources will be shown in an appropriate way throughout the study.

Pass (50–69 marks)

The study will include a systematic review of relevant literature or other sources of information or data. There may be some evidence of originality in the research question(s) or in the approach taken to the subject. The research will contain a synthesis of appropriate ideas, evidence or data. Good use will be made of data and information to highlight new knowledge, to support argument, or to criticise current ideas, approaches, research methods or practices.

The discussion of methods and sources will include arguments in support of the methods or approach taken, or a description of the project design. There will be some references to the research methods literature or similar appropriate material. An attempt will be made to reflect on the research method used.

The dissertation will be well structured and written in good English. Accurate referencing of sources will be shown in the appropriate way.

Fail (49 marks or under)

The research question(s) will not be well developed. There will be a limited review of appropriate literature or sources of information or data. The dissertation will contain an incomplete or sketchy treatment of theoretical or empirical material. The development of the data or information collected will be descriptive and may not be used in the right way. Argument is less likely to be developed or sustained.

Discussion of research methods will not be developed and is likely to contain important errors. There will be a lack of judgement about the research method used.

The dissertation will be poorly written. Referencing will be generally inaccurate or inadequate.

2. Degree of difficulty

The degree of difficulty of the research attempted needs to be distinguished. This can be done in combination with the description (aspect 1 above) and the key words (aspect 3 below) by judgement of *one or more* of the following four criteria:

(a) the degree of difficulty contained within the research question(s);
(b) the degree of difficulty contained in the methodology;
(c) the degree of difficulty in synthesis and the organisation of the research findings;
(d) the degree of difficulty in the evidence collected or arguments presented.

3. Key words

Distinction	Pass	Fail
accuracy	analysis	brief
ambition	application	description
appraisal	calculation	error
balance	demonstration	incomplete
critical	experiment	irrelevant
evaluation	ideas	narrow
evidence	knowledge	omission
imagination	organisation	superficiality
interpretation	reflection	vagueness
judgement	review	
originality	sources	
rigorous	structure	
scope	synthesis	
style		
testing		
theory		

Note to students: Distinction level should also include criteria of the Pass category (in aspect 3 above).

Summary

This chapter explained the role of the supervisor and the importance of planning your research to achieve the desired outcome. In short, your supervisor will provide you with the appropriate direction towards the production of your dissertation. He/she can advise you on the research strategy, methodology and structure of your dissertation. Your supervisor is not obliged to proofread or correct spelling and grammar.

It is essential that you time-manage your work. Therefore, drawing up a realistic work schedule is highly recommended.

It is also important to keep in close contact with your supervisor. You should arrange a formal meeting with him/her at least three times throughout the whole process.

Finally, it is also recommended to keep the log form up to date in order to record your progress.

Reference

Buckley, M and Naoum, S. (2011) *Dissertation Guide: Instructions for Preparation, Control and Presentation of the Dissertation*. Department of Property, Surveying and Construction, London South Bank University.

Appendix 1
Examples of dissertation proposals

Proposal 1: proposal for a descriptive type of research

Working title

Marketing and the private house-building companies: which marketing philosophy do successful companies have?

Rationale

The subject of this proposal developed from a personal interest in the dichotomy between technical excellence and customer orientation. In their book *In Search of Excellence*, Peters and Waterman[1] point out that the most successful US firms were characterised by a common dedication to marketing. More specifically the key to success lies in 'keeping close to the customer'.

The size of private housing market in relation to total construction output is rather significant. It accounts for 14 per cent of construction output for an all work total and 24 per cent of construction output for total new work.[2] Hence, the proposed study is an important one and the author will be focusing on the marketing philosophy of the private house-building companies.

Literature provides numerous alternative definitions of marketing; most have certain basic features in common, especially the notion of looking at the firm from the point of view of the customer or striving to ensure mutual profitability from the marketing exchange. Other definitions place the emphasis on the essential managerial nature of marketing. Marketing, however, should be distinguished from selling.[3] Selling is only one of several marketing functions and may not be the most important.[4] In addition, selling may require a different set of skills from those needed for marketing.[5]

Another important aspect of marketing which deserves close attention is 'Relational Marketing'. The marketing-led enterprise change management initiated by a major UK contractor was explored by Smyth and Fitch[6] in their paper titled 'Application of relationship marketing and management: a large contractor case study'. Their premise was that procurement-led initiatives try to induce changes to behaviour through market governance. In their abstract, they stated:

Relationship marketing and management proactively change organizational behaviour, the enterprise taking responsibility for its own destiny. Investment and resource allocation, and organizational behaviour have posed constraints, particularly concerning service continuity in construction. Relationship marketing is the conceptual starting point, application developing into relationship management in line with theory. In the case explored, key account management (KAM) principles are adopted as the conceptual point of departure for introducing relationship marketing processes. Adoption resulted in some minor restructuring and provided the basis for a series of process changes. Application is producing early results in terms of increased client satisfaction, consequential repeat business, inducing greater cross-functional communication and collaboration within the firm resulting in cross-selling opportunities between market segments. Some repeat business is producing higher margins in response to meeting demands of the clients.

The principal theme of this research is to use Stanton and Futrell's[7] marketing profiles and place each of the companies to be studied in a particular category and then link it to its financial performance. Stanton and Futrell established three marketing profile categories, namely, Production Orientation, Sales Orientation and Marketing Orientation.

The following sections of this proposal give further details about the principal objectives for this research.

Research goals

Aim

To construct a reference table that demonstrates those marketing philosophies of private house-building that led to a high financial performance.

Objectives

1 To survey large private house-building companies and investigate the following:
   (a) their business philosophy
   (b) organisational structure
   (c) marketing information system
   (d) marketing planning and policy.
2 To explore companies' views concerning the philosophy of relational marketing.
3 To test the relationship between the companies' marketing philosophy and their financial performance.

Key questions

1 How do private house-building companies differ in marketing their businesses?
2 How do different private house-building companies view relational marketing?
3 Which marketing philosophy leads to higher financial performance?

Hypothesis

1 Most private house-building companies adopt the 'sales oriented' philosophy.
2 Relational marketing can increase client satisfaction.
3 Private house-building companies that adopt a 'high relational marketing' perform better financially.

Note to students: Notice that in this proposal, the student formulated 3 objectives, 3 key questions and 3 hypotheses. They are all interlinked in such a way that objective 1 is related to key question 1 and to hypothesis 1. Objective 2 is related to key question 2 and to hypothesis 2, and so on.

Initial literature review

In this part of the proposal, the student provided a two-page initial literature review about the subject of 'marketing'. This part of the proposal is basically an extension of the Rationale section given above. Do not forget to supplement your initial literature with supporting empirical facts that are fully referenced.

Methodology

Note to students: In this section of the proposal you need to draw the methodology road map related to your research as shown in the example in Figure 2.3 and Figure 9.2.

Below is an outline of the stages involved

Stage 1: literature review

This study will be confined to the private house-building sector, where there is a more direct link between the company and the end user. The initial survey of the literature reveals no specific study of marketing in the private house-building industry. However, the desk work for this study will concentrate on research which has looked at the construction industry in general, such as the earlier research of O'Callaghan[7] and Stilgoe.[8] This should provide a useful point of reference.

Stage 2: pilot study

Data collection will take the form of a structured postal questionnaire. However, an initial pilot study will be conducted to test the validity of the questionnaire through in-depth interviews with marketing managers.

Stage 3: main survey questionnaire

The feedback from the pilot study should assist in finalising the questionnaire and preparing the ground for the main survey. The questions will centre around the areas mentioned in the above objectives. In order to obtain a high level of response, a multi-option format will be designed and limited to about 30 questions. Open questions are considered to be inappropriate as they would require the respondents to formulate an answer which needs lengthier input and will therefore be more difficult to analyse.

Stage 4: analysing the postal questionnaire

The analysis of the questionnaire will take two forms. First, to determine the level of agreement or disagreement of the respondents to each question within the questionnaire by counting the number of respondents who answered favourably or unfavourably. Judging by the response, each company will be placed in one of the three marketing profile categories, that is Production Orientation, Sales Orientation or Marketing Orientation. Second, to correlate each of the marketing philosophy questions to the financial performance of each company. Financial information will be obtained from the business ratio report and from companies' annual reports. The level of financial performance will be gauged by establishing a marketing rating system applicable to private house-building companies.

Stage 5: writing the research report

This stage involves writing up the content of the dissertation and should cover the chapters proposed in the following section.

Proposed structure of the dissertation

Chapter 1: Introduction
Chapter 2: Marketing theory and principles
Chapter 3: Marketing and the construction industry
Chapter 4: Research design and methodology
Chapter 5: Analysis of the results and discussion
Chapter 6: Conclusions and suggestions for further research
Chapter 7: References

Initial references

1 Peters, T.Z. and Waterman, R.H. (1982) *In Search of Excellence: Lessons from America's Best Run Companies*. New York: Harper and Row.
2 National Economic Development Office (2010) *Construction Forecast 2010–2011–2012*. London: HMSO.
3 Foster, D. (1984) *Mastering Marketing*. Hong Kong: Macmillan.
4 Kotler, P. and Armstrong, G. (1996) *Principles of Marketing*. Seventh edition. Prentice Hall, Inc.
5 Fisher, N. (1986) *Marketing for the Construction Industry*. London: Longman.
6 Smyth, H. and Fitch, T. (2009) Application of relationship marketing and management: a large contractor case study. *Construction Management and Economics*, 27(4), 399–410.
7 Stanton, W. and Futrell, C. (1986) *Fundamentals of Marketing*. International edition. New York: McGraw-Hill.
8 O'Callaghan, J. (1986) Managerial Characteristics and Financial Performance of Construction Companies. MSc thesis, Brunel University.
9 Stilgoe, G. (1985) 'Marketing policy and construction firms.' MSc dissertation, Brunel University.

Programme of work

In this section of the proposal, a bar chart or a breakdown of activities, like the one shown in Figure 10.1, should be attached showing the programme of work for the dissertation. It should also indicate the target dates for the completion of each of the stages shown in the methodology section.

Proposal 2: proposal for the analytical approach/ theoretical framework

Working title

The influence of procurement method on project performance: a comparative study between management contracting and the traditional form of contracts.

Rationale

It is axiomatic of construction management that a project may be regarded as successful if the building is delivered at the right time, at the appropriate price and quality standard, as well as achieving a high level of client satisfaction. Increasingly, the achievement of these criteria has been associated with the method of procurement. In short, the selection of the appropriate method can shape the success of the project and this research has chosen to study the performance of management contracting and traditional contracting.

The problems associated with the building process have always been considered in relation to separation of design from construction (Latham, 1994; Egan, 1997) and lack of integration (Sidwell, 1979), poor communication (Higgins *et al.*, 1965; Doloi, 2009) and increasing project complexity (Bennett *et al.*, 1980). These factors, together with economic changes, for example inflation and recession (Hillebrandt, 1985), have led construction professionals and the industry to offer alternative methods of procurement, such as management contracting, design and build and project management.

With the growth in the use of these methods in the mid-1970s, a number of researchers have investigated the management of the building process and in particular the performance in terms of time, cost and quality. In one study, the relationship between contractual arrangement and project success was investigated on 32 building projects, from which it was found that the essential element which brought about success was the level of managerial control (Sidwell, 1982). Of the contractual methods studied, those with a high level of managerial control, for example management contracting, performed better on time, gave a high level of client satisfaction and overran the budget by less.

The case study approach has been used previously to illustrate the performance of management contracting, but either the results were based on small samples or the number of management contracts studied were very limited. Moreover, there have been relatively few investigations which have analysed the characteristics of the client, the designer and project within the scope of one study.

Research goals

Aim

To construct a scoring matrix showing the level of performance between management and traditional form of contracts.

Objectives

1 To establish the background, apparent advantages and disadvantages to the client in adopting management and traditional contracting.
2 To evaluate the client criteria and priority when selecting management contracting.
3 To find out whether the characteristics of the client have a significant effect on project performance.
4 To find out whether the characteristics of the project have a significant effect on project performance.
5 To compare the performance of time and cost of commercial projects completed under management and traditional contracts.

Key research questions

1 How would the client benefit from selecting the new procurement route of management contracting and what are its shortfalls?
2 What would be the main criteria used by clients to choose management contracting for their future commercial projects?
3 To what extent does the experience of the client with the building process have an effect on project success?
4 To what extent does the characteristic of the project have an effect on project success?
5 How did commercial projects perform, in terms of time and cost, under management contracting compared with similar projects built using the traditional form contract?

Theoretical argument

The theory that I will use will be the contingency theory. It was developed by Kast and Rosenzweig (1973) and it was used to study the management of organisation, including organisation design, leadership, behavioural change and operations. The contingency theory indicates that there is no one way to design, manage or to organise a business enterprise; it is contingent or dependent upon the problem or situation in hand (independent variables). As applied to my study, this theory will hold that I would expect my independent variables (client and project characteristics) to influence the intervening variable (procurement method) and in turn influence the dependent variable (project performance). This proposition is thought to apply to my research because the contingency approach recognises the complexity involved in managing modern organisations, but uses the pattern of relationships and/or configurations of subsystems in order to facilitate improved practice.

The research hypotheses

Based on the above theoretical argument and the literature review, the following hypotheses are formulated:

Main hypothesis

'In order to achieve a high level of project performance, the procurement method should be selected in accordance to the characteristics of the client and the project.'

This main hypothesis can be broken down into the following sub-hypotheses:

1 Management contracting has certain advantages to offer but also has some shortfalls.
2 Management contracting can be best used when time is of the essence.
3 Management contracting can be best used for inexperienced clients.
4 Management contracting can be best used for highly complex projects.
5 Traditional contacts are more likely to deliver projects within budget when compared with similar projects delivered under management contracting.

Note to students: Notice that in this proposal, the author formulated five objects, five key questions, five sub-hypotheses. They are all interlinked in such a way that objective 1 is related to key question 1 and to hypothesis 1. Objective 2 is related to key question 2 and to hypothesis 2, and so on.

Initial literature review

Note to students: In this part of the proposal, the author provided a two-page initial literature about the subject of 'procurement methods'. This part of the proposal is basically an extension of the Rationale section given above. Do not forget to supplement your initial literature with supporting empirical facts that are fully referenced.

Outline methodology

The methodology road map related to this research is shown in Figure 9.2 and below is an outline of the stages involved.

Stage 1: literature review

This study will first review the relevant literature on the subject of procurement methods, in particular, looking at previous building process models which studied the performance of the procurement method. For example, the work of Sidwell (1982) is particularly relevant.

The main sources of information will be the following: ARCOM Abstract (www.arcom.ac.uk/abstracts.html), ASCE, CME, ECAM, IPM Journals and previous dissertations and PhD theses.

Stage 2: designing the research framework/model

It is the author's intention to modify and update the theoretical framework shown in Figure 9.2 (stage 2). This will be used to test relationships and associations among the variables using case studies.

Stage 3: constructing the questionnaire

The literature review and the design of the theoretical framework will be followed by constructing a data collection questionnaire which will be used to compare the performance of management and traditional contracts.

It is intended to adopt the quantitative data collection approach, which means obtaining facts and figures from previously completed projects in addition to obtaining opinions and views of those involved in the project. It is also intended to obtain a large sample of cases, approximately 60 projects, all of which will be analysed statistically. (Table 6.2 is an extract from Naoum's questionnaire.)

Stage 4: the pilot study

As recommended by previous writers, this research will conduct a pilot study before collecting the final data from the whole sample. This should provide a trial run for the questionnaire of stage 3 above, which involves testing the wording of the questions, identifying ambiguous questions, testing the technique that I will use to collect the data, measuring the effectiveness of my standard invitation to respondents and so on.

The author's pilot study will take the form of structured interviews with two clients and two contractors who have commissioned and experienced 'pure' management projects. An interview questionnaire will be used for this pilot study in order to validate the appropriateness of the main study questionnaire.

Stage 5: the main study

The pilot study should prepare the ground for modifying the main study questionnaire which will be used to compare the performance of management and traditional contracts.

The inferential statistical tests will be applied. It will consist of hypotheses testing, tables of correlation and association and interpretation of the results. The tables will show whether there are significant differences in time, cost, quality and safety performance between management contracting and the traditional form of contracts.

Stage 6: writing up

This stage involves writing up the content of the dissertation and should cover the chapters proposed in the following section.

Proposed structure of dissertation

Chapter 1: Introduction and background to the problem
Chapter 2: Review of the traditional and management contracting
Chapter 3: Review of previous models of the building process
Chapter 4: Research design and method of analysis
Chapter 5: Analysis of the results
Chapter 6: Conclusions
Chapter 7: References

Initial references

Bennett, J. and Fine, B. (1980) *Measurement of Complexity in Construction Projects.* Reading: Department of Construction Management, University of Reading.

Doloi, H (2009) Relational partnerships: the importance of communication, trust and confidence and joint risk management in achieving project success. *Construction Management and Economics*, 27(11), 1099–1109.

Egan Report (1997) *Rethinking Construction: Report of the Construction Task Force.* London: HMSO.

Higgin, G. and Jessop, N. (1965) *Communication in the Building Industry.* London: Tavistock Institute.

Hillebrandt, P. (1977) *Economic Theory and the Construction Industry.* London: Macmillan.

Kast, F. and Rosenzweig, V. (1973) *Contingency Views of Organisation and Management.* London: Science Research Associates.

Latham Report (1994) *Constructing the Team.* London: HMSO.

Sidwell, A. (1979) *A Field Study of Organisational Forms.* Birmingham: Department of Construction and Environmental Health, University of Aston.

Sidwell, A. (1982) 'A critical study of project team organisational forms within the building process', PhD thesis, Department of Construction and Environmental Health, University of Aston.

Research programme

In this section of the proposal, a bar chart or a breakdown of activities, like the one shown in Figure 10.1, should be attached showing the programme of work for the dissertation. It should also indicate the target dates for the completion of each of the stages shown in the methodology section.

Proposal 3: proposal for the problem-solving approach

Working title

An evaluation of the total quality management system: a case study.

Rationale

The problem of quality and its associated costs has been of great concern to most industries since the early 1960s. As a result, some large construction contractors have pursued and implemented innovative quality management techniques such as quality assurance (QA) and total quality management (TQM). Oakland (1990) defined TQM as a way of managing to improve the effectiveness, flexibility and competitiveness of a business as a whole. It applies just as much to service industries as it does to manufacturing. It involves whole companies getting organised in every department, every activity and every person at every level.

Once management acknowledges that there is a problem, it can take the second step to develop a clear understanding of underlying principles and elements of TQM such as training (Imai and Kaisen, 1986), team work (Aubrey and Felkins, 1988), supplier involvement, customer services and its implementation, which is considered by Juran (1988) as the primary quality management tool.

According to Boardman and Croxson (1994), several senior TQM representatives from various client and contracting organisations forming the European Construction Institute TQM Task Force were discussing this very topic of measuring, where their companies were on the TQM journey, and it became manifestly obvious that there were various methods for the measurement of TQM. The preliminary literature review revealed that Boardman's measurement chart is simple but comprehensive and can be used to give a visual representation of the organisation's current position in a TQM programme.

Based on such a background, this research will be using the matrix model developed by the Trafalgar House Quality Management Services organisation as the tool to identify the specific problems within the author's organisation and to make recommendations, if appropriate, for improving the quality system.

Aim

To propose a guideline for implementing a total quality management system for large contracting organisations.

Objectives

1   To review the concept and principle of TQM.
2   To assess the advantages of the TQM systems.
3   To measure the efficiency of the current quality management system in the author's organisation and to identify any present problems within the system.

4   To design and recommend a new TQM system for the organisation.
5   To evaluate the proposed TQM.

Hypothesis

Note to students: With the problem-solving approach, formulating a hypothesis is not usually applicable. It is applicable only when the proposed solution is to be put under test, which is not practical at undergraduate level. Instead, a number of key questions can be formed.

Key questions

1   What are the reasons that drive the construction industry towards accreditation of standard QA?
2   Does accreditation of QA assure the customer of an optimum standard of services?
3   What are the differences between QA and total TQM?

Methodology

Note to students: Here you need to draw the methodology road map related to your research as shown in the example in Figure 2.3 and Figure 9.2.

Below is an outline of the stages involved

Stage 1: literature research

A comprehensive review of the relevant literature including a computer-assisted search will be undertaken in order to develop an understanding of previous work in the field of TQM.

Stage 2: exploratory interviews

This stage will explore the matrix designed by the Trafalgar House Quality Management Services House. The exploration will be achieved through unstructured interviews with five companies that are known to have implemented a TQM system.

Stage 3: case study

The author will then use his or her own organisation as a case to study the possible implementation of a systematic TQM. Interviews with employees will take place to score the level of quality effectiveness.

Stage 4: evaluation of the organisation's present TQM system

This stage will bring together and review the information collected in the previous stages in which the present TQM system has to be studied.

Stage 5: writing up

This stage involves writing up the content of the dissertation and should cover the chapters proposed in the following section.

Proposed contents of dissertation

Chapter 1: Introduction
Chapter 2: Total quality management – the concept
Chapter 3: Implementation of TQM
Chapter 4: Designing the case study and research methodology
Chapter 5: Analysing and evaluating the case study evidence
Chapter 6: Conclusions and further studies
Chapter 7: References

Initial references

Aubrey, C. and Felkins, P. (1988) *Teamwork: Involving People in Quality and Productivity Improvement*. Milwaukee: American Society of Quality Control.

Boardman, R. and Croxson, J. (1994) *Trafalgar Quality Management Services*. Unpublished report by the Trafalgar House Company, UK, 25 pages.

Imai, M. and Kaisen, L. (1986) *The Key to Japan's Competitive Success*. New York: Random House.

Juran, J. (1988) *Juran on Planning for Quality*. New York: The Free Press.

Oakland, J. (1990) *Total Quality Management*. Oxford: Butterworth-Heinemann.

Programme of work

In this section of the proposal, a bar chart or a breakdown of activities, like the one shown in Figure 10.1, should be attached showing the programme of work for the dissertation. It should also indicate the target dates for the completion of each of the stages shown in the methodology section.

Proposal 4: proposal for the desk study approach – analysis of secondary source of data

Working title

Safety and the construction industry: a statistical analysis of facts and figures of the safety record during boom and bust of the construction industry.

Rationale

In the construction industry, the risk of a fatality is five times more likely than in a manufacturing-based industry, whereas the risk of a major injury is two and a half times higher. A Health and Safety Executive study (HSE, 2007) reveals that construction has one of the highest ratios of non-injury to injury accidents of all UK industries. Apart from the human cost of suffering an accident, the economic effect can be devastating. Direct costs of accidents such as injury, illness or damage can be insured against, although this is the tip of a very large iceberg. Every £1 of an accident costs that an insurance company has to pay out could cost the contractor between £5 and £50 in indirect costs. These indirect costs will range from product and material damage to legal costs (Travers Morgan Ltd, 1995).

Therefore, the Health and Safety Executive has, for many years, sought to promote a business case for health and safety management, including highlighting the downside costs of poor management such as lost time, lost productivity and fines as well as the business benefits, such as increased profits (Antonelli *et al.*, 2006).

A better health and safety (H&S) management would help reduce accidents, which would eliminate damage to equipment, machinery and raw materials. This in turn leads to an increase of output to firms and thereby lead to higher output in the economy. Naoum and colleagues (2010) suggest that safer work conditions and healthier workers may increase the productivity of labour hours and thereby contribute to higher productivity and output.

Wright and colleagues (2005) state that 'evidence that good health and safety improves productivity' is the top ranked incentive for improving health and safety. It is further reported by Shearn (2003) that 10 per cent of UK businesses will be prepared to increase their effort in H&S management, if they are provided with evidence that it would result in 'business benefits'. These benefits include a mix of both tangible and intangible benefits, such as maintenance of reputation, client requirements, controlling insurance premium costs and reduction in absence rates as well as general improvements in health and safety (Antonelli *et al.*, 2006). To compound this point, research by McCon (1997) has suggested that in firms that have demonstrated good, sustained safety performance, you will usually find the added benefits of good housekeeping, good product quality and high morale

Despite the many ethical and moral reasons to invest in H&S, organisations seem motivated to improve aspects of H&S because of the potential risk to the business if H&S is not addressed. Research by Antonelli and colleagues (2006) concluded that although some organisations are convinced of carrying out H&S initiatives, this tends to be driven by the need to manage costs (mainly insurance premiums) or by demands made by customers (to ensure they are eligible to participate in tendering processes, and also to maintain existing business), or by the risk of being non-compliant and the adverse effects this may have on the prospect of winning new business.

Unfortunately, to date, evaluations of H&S activities have tended to focus on H&S-based performance metrics such as injury rates. Little attention has been given to the economic contributions and impacts that H&S may bring. There appears to have been few coordinated attempts to identify and assess the full spectrum of potential economic benefits and impacts, both to individual organisations and to the UK economy.

According to Smallman (2001), almost no scientific base was found for supporting the assertion that there is a business case for investment in H&S, in other words, that such investment produces returns to stakeholders. The little evidence that exists is based largely around anecdote, which claims that excellence in H&S does produce returns, and mainly from reduced insurance premiums. Notwithstanding this, whereas the economic and moral cases for investment in H&S are indisputable, the argument that 'safety pays', frequently used by government, is spurious.

Research goals

Aim

To analyse historical HSE statistics and find out whether there is a link between the economic climate and the rate of accidents in the construction industry.

Objectives

1 To provide a general overview of the history of accidents in the construction industry before and after the introduction of the CDM [Construction (Design and Managenent)] regulations.
2 To analyse the ratio of accidents to employees in order to find out the trades with the highest accident rate.
3 To analyse the cost and benefits of implementing safety policies by the contractors.
4 To find out whether there is a correlation between the state of the general economy and the rate of accidents.

Key questions

1 How did different contractors respond to the CDM regulation?
2 What is the ratio of accidents to number of employees in the UK construction industry compared with the manufacturing industry?
3 How much would companies benefit from having a H&S policy?
4 To what extent would safety in construction be affected by the state of the economy and vice versa?

Assumptions

1 CDM regulations are applied in the construction industry as a force rather than a belief.
2 Accident rates in construction are twice as high as in the manufacturing industry.
3 The benefits of investing in safety outweigh the cost by more than eight times.
4 Productivity rate can be an accurate indicator for measuring the link between safety and the economic climate.

Note to students: Notice that in this proposal, the student formulated four objects, four key questions, four assumptions. They are all interlinked in such a way that objective 1 is related to key question 1 and to assumption 1. Objective 2 is related to key question 2 and to assumption 2, and so on.

Methodology

Note to students: Here you need to draw the methodology road map related to your research as shown in the example in Figure 2.3 and Figure 9.2.

Below is an outline of the stages involved

Stage 1: literature review

The basic concern throughout the review stage is to identify some of the broader parameters likely to be relevant in studying the construction industry's safety statistics. In order to achieve the first objective, a systematic literature review is to be conducted which will cover textbooks, institutional and statutory publications, periodicals and trade/academic journals, seminar and conference papers. In particular, the following sources will be cited:

- The Loughborough University Research
- HSE report No. CRR229/1999
- HSE report No. CD 207

Stage 2: analysing the facts and figures

The second objective of the study can be achieved by analysing published and unpublished accident statistical data, which will be acquired from the Health and Safety Statistical Services Department in Liverpool.

The third objective will be achieved by gathering information from the Health and Safety Executive Report entitled *Cost Benefits of Implementing the CDM Regulations 2007*. This objective will show how the distribution of accident costs affect the industry and society.

To achieve the fourth objective, information about the economic climate during the last decade will be gathered from the HMSO construction output and then correlated with the accident record, in an attempt to find out whether the rate of accidents is related to recession. The statistical package SPSS will be utilised to assist in evaluating this relationship.

Stage 3: producing tables and graphs to present the results

Note to students: This is part of the writing-up stage in which all the results will be presented in graphical format to allow discussion and interpretation to be made on the research findings.

Proposed structure of dissertation

Chapter 1: Introduction to the safety problem
Chapter 2: Health and safety and the employment trend
Chapter 3: Safety culture in the construction industry
Chapter 4: Previous empirical research on construction safety
Chapter 5: Analysis of the secondary data
Chapter 6: Discussion and critical appraisal
Chapter 7: Conclusion and recommendation for further research
Chapter 8: References

Initial references

Antonelli, A., Baker, M., McMahon, A. and Wright, M. (2006) Six SME Case Studies that Demonstrate the Business Benefit of Effective Health and Safety Management: Contract Research Report 504, Prepared by Green Street Berman for HSE, HMSO, London.

Barnard, M. (1995) 'Safety is the Engineers Responsibility: Facts or Fiction?' A paper given by the Director of Health and Safety for Travers Morgan Ltd at the Institute of Civil Engineers on Construction Site Safety and the CDM regulations, 6 February, School of Business and Industrial Management.

Construction News (1994) Preparing for Safety Laws. *Construction News,* 1 December, p. 16.

Davies, V. and Tomasin, K. (1990) *Construction Site Safety.* London: Thomas Telford.

HSE (Health and Safety Executive) (1983) *The Costs of Accidents at Work.* London: Health and Safety Commission, HMSO.

HSE (2007) *Managing Health Safety in Construction, Construction (Design and Management) Regulations 2007, Approved Code of Practice and Guidance.* London: HMSO.

McCon, P. (1997) Housekeeping & Injury Rate: A Correlation Study. *Professional Safety,* December, pp. 29–32.

Naoum, S., Hemmings, B. and D. Fong (2011) 'Is there a correlation between contractor's health and safety performance and their profit margins?' 6th International Structural Engineering and Construction Conference (ISEC – 6), 21–26 June, Zurich. Paper ID S1-C32.

Shearn, P. (2004). *Workforce Participation in the Management of Occupational Health & Safety*. Health & Safety Executive Report No. ERG/04/01, London.

Smallman, C. (2001) The Reality of 'Revitalizing Health and Safety'. *Journal of Safety Research*, 32, 391–439. Travers Morgan Ltd (1995) 'The Economics of Safety Management'. A paper given by Mr Mike Crocker of Travers Morgan Ltd at Walfords, London.

Wright, M., Antonelli, A., Doyle, J.N., Bendig, M., and Genna, R. (2005) 'An evidence based evaluation of how best to secure compliance with health and safety law', Health and Safety Executive Research Report 334. Suffolk: HSE Books.

Proposed programme of work

In this section of the proposal, a bar chart or a breakdown activities, like the one shown in Figure 10.1, should be attached showing the programme of work for the dissertation. It should also indicate the target dates for the completion of each of the stages shown in the methodology section.

Appendix 2
London South Bank
University: example of a
questionnaire

MARKETING QUESTIONNAIRE

Please respond to the following questions by either ticking the appropriate box or writing your answer in the space provided.

Please note: All information provided will be treated in the strictest of confidence.

Section 1 – questions related to company details

1.1 Please indicate the approximate turnover of your practice

Less than £2m	£2.1–6m	£6.1–10m	More than £10m (Please state)
☐	☐	☐	_____

1.2 What percentage of this is attributed specifically to marketing (approximately)?

Less than 1%	1–2%	3–5%	More than 5% (Please state)
☐	☐	☐	_____

1.3 Does the practice have a separate marketing department? YES ☐ NO ☐

IF YES

A. How many people are employed in this department? Please tick appropriate box.

1–2	3–5	6–8	More than 8 (Please state)
☐	☐	☐	_____

B. How long has this marketing department been established? Please tick.

0–2 years   3–4 years   5–6 years   More than 6 years
(Please state)

☐   ☐   ☐   _____

IF NO

Please tick one box to indicate for what reasons.

– A marketing department is not considered necessary   ☐

– The practice is too small to employ individuals for this   ☐

– Marketing tends to be a management role   ☐

– Other (please specify)   ☐

_____

_____

_____

1.4 What does the practice perceive as its future marketing trend over the next 5 years?

– To decrease   ☐

– To remain stable   ☐

– To increase   ☐

1.5 Which statement best describes your organisational philosophy? Please tick one box.

– To achieve modest growth   ☐

– To achieve a greater share of the market place   ☐

– To achieve service and quality   ☐

Section 2 – questions related to marketing strategy and policy

2.1 What level of priority is given to marketing within your business strategy? Please tick one box.

– High priority   ☐

– Moderate priority   ☐

– Low priority   ☐

2.2 Which statement best describes the role of marketing within your practice? Please tick one box.

– It is perceived to be the role of upper management   ☐

– Marketing plays a role with all our staff ☐

– It is left to the marketing department/key individuals ☐

2.3 Which statement best describes the way in which your practice is driven? Please tick one box.

– Technology driven ☐

– Customer driven ☐

– Market driven ☐

2.4 Are planning and operations within departments orientated towards customer satisfaction? Please tick one box.

– Yes, very much so ☐

– Yes, in some departments ☐

– No, other factors dominate ☐

2.5 Which statement best describes the way your practice allocates its resources to a project? Please tick one box.

– Resources are governed by the fee and required profit ☐

– Governed by the client's actual requirements ☐

– Governed by the type of client (i.e. new client etc.) ☐

2.6 Is training given to your staff on the basics of marketing? Please tick one or more box(es).

– Yes, we undertake regular training sessions ☐

– We have in the past given staff training ☐

– No, we have never given any formal training ☐

2.7 Does your marketing department seek advice from outside PR agencies?

YES ☐ NO ☐

If Yes, for how long? _____ Yrs

If No, for what reasons? (Please specify) _____

_____

_____

_____

Section 3 – questions related to the marketing techniques

3.1 From the following marketing and promotional techniques please indicate which techniques your firm practises by stating yes/no. If yes, how important do you consider them in making clients aware of your firm?

Marketing/ promotional techniques	Do you use? Yes/No	← Not important/very important →				
		1	2	3	4	5
Company brochure						
Company newsletter						
Seminars						
Presentations						
Videos						
Entertaining						
Advertising through media						
Other forms of advertising (i.e. site boards etc.)						
Introduction letter						
Company logo						

3.2   If your practice was presenting itself to a client which statement would best describe the initial approach it would use to sell itself? Please tick box(es)

– We would concentrate on past projects, with emphasis on experience and reputation ☐

– We would focus on the particular client's needs, relative to the project ☐

– We would promote the technical facilities and capabilities of the practice ☐

– We would promote value for money and cost ☐

3.3   How often does your practice thoroughly research a new client and the services they require? Please tick box(es) ☐

– We attempt to do this for all clients ☐

– We do research, but not as much as we should ☐

– We tend to offer our own range of services first ☐

3.4   Which statement best describes the primary objectives of your marketing strategy? ☐

– To achieve increased market share and new clients ☐

– Service excellence is our primary objective ☐

– Technical excellence and expertise should be exploited ☐

Section 4 – questions related to the selection process

4.1   In making initial contact with a client, how influential are the following? Please tick appropriate cell.

Forms of initial contact	← Least influential/most influential →				
	1	2	3	4	5
Advertisements	___	___	___	___	___
Recommendations	___	___	___	___	___
Introduction letters/portfolios	___	___	___	___	___
Industry reputation	___	___	___	___	___
Previous working relationships	___	___	___	___	___
Contacts	___	___	___	___	___
Following leads	___	___	___	___	___
Others (please state and rank):	___	___	___	___	___
_____	___	___	___	___	___
_____	___	___	___	___	___

4.2   How important do you consider the following criteria when being selected by a client for your services? Please tick appropriate cell.

CRITERION	Little importance	Some importance	Quite important	Important	Very important
Turnover/size of practice					
Status/market share					
Financial standing/ stability					
Technical capability/ excellence					
Quality of personnel and expertise					
Obtaining/having QA					
Being chartered					
Experience					

Professional reputation/track record						
Prior business relationships/ clients						
Lowest price/fees						
Presentation						
Previous projects (type)						
Range of services offered						
Geographical location						
Attention to detail						
Company offices and general image						
Negotiating skill						
Informal contacts						
Responsiveness						

Section 5 – general questions

5.1   What are the main hurdles/problems in reaching a client? Please give brief details.

_____

_____

_____

5.2   Do you feel there is any way QS Practices can improve the services they offer (if necessary)?

_____

_____

_____

Thank you for your participation, please send the completed questionnaires in the self-addressed envelope provided.

Appendix 3
Statistical tables

Table A *Distribution of t*

df	Probability					
	0.5	0.1	0.05	0.02	0.01	0.001
1	1.000	6.314	12.706	31.821	63.657	636.619
2	0.816	2.920	4.303	6.965	9.925	31.598
3	0.765	2.353	3.182	4.541	5.841	12.941
4	0.741	2.132	2.776	3.747	4.604	8.610
5	0.727	2.015	2.571	3.365	4.032	6.859
6	0.718	1.943	2.447	3.143	3.707	5.959
7	0.711	1.895	2.365	2.998	3.499	5.405
8	0.706	1.860	2.306	2.896	3.355	5.041
9	0.703	1.833	2.262	2.821	3.250	4.781
10	0.700	1.812	2.228	2.764	3.169	4.587
11	0.697	1.796	2.201	2.718	3.106	4.437
12	0.695	1.782	2.179	2.681	3.055	4.318
13	0.694	1.771	2.160	2.650	3.012	4.221
14	0.692	1.761	2.145	2.624	2.977	4.140
15	0.691	1.753	2.131	2.602	2.947	4.073
16	0.690	1.746	2.120	2.583	2.921	4.015
17	0.689	1.740	2.110	2.567	2.898	3.965
18	0.688	1.734	2.101	2.552	2.878	3.922
19	0.688	1.729	2.093	2.539	2.861	3.883
20	0.687	1.725	2.086	2.528	2.845	3.850
21	0.686	1.721	2.080	2.518	2.831	3.819
22	0.686	1.717	2.074	2.508	2.819	3.792
23	0.685	1.714	2.069	2.500	2.807	3.767
24	0.685	1.711	2.064	2.492	2.797	3.745
25	0.684	1.708	2.060	2.485	2.787	3.725
26	0.684	1.706	2.056	2.479	2.779	3.707
27	0.684	1.703	2.052	2.473	2.771	3.690
28	0.683	1.701	2.048	2.467	2.763	3.674
29	0.683	1.699	2.045	2.462	2.756	3.659
30	0.683	1.697	2.042	2.457	2.750	3.646
40	0.681	1.684	2.021	2.423	2.704	3.551
60	0.679	1.671	2.000	2.390	2.660	3.460
120	0.677	1.658	1.980	2.358	2.617	3.373
∝	0.674	1.645	1.960	2.326	2.576	3.291

Source: Adapted by permission of the authors and publishers from Table III (Fisher and Yates, 1974).

Table B   *Distribution of χ^2*

df	Probability					
	0.5	0.1	0.05	0.02	0.01	0.001
1	0.455	2.706	3.841	5.412	6.635	10.827
2	1.386	4.605	5.991	7.824	9.210	13.815
3	2.366	6.251	7.815	9.837	11.345	16.268
4	3.357	7.779	9.488	11.668	13.277	18.465
5	4.351	9.236	11.070	13.388	15.086	20.517
6	5.348	10.645	12.592	15.033	16.812	22.457
7	6.346	12.017	14.067	16.622	18.475	24.322
8	7.344	13.362	15.507	18.168	20.090	26.125
9	8.343	14.684	16.919	19.679	21.666	28.877
10	9.342	15.987	18.307	21.161	23.209	29.588
11	10.341	17.275	19.675	22.618	24.725	31.264
12	11.340	18.549	21.026	24.054	26.217	32.909
13	12.340	19.812	22.362	25.472	27.688	34.528
14	13.339	21.064	23.685	26.873	29.141	36.123
15	14.339	22.307	24.996	28.259	30.578	37.697
16	15.338	23.542	26.296	29.633	32.000	39.252
17	16.338	24.769	27.587	30.995	33.409	40.790
18	17.338	25.989	28.869	32.346	34.805	42.321
19	18.338	27.204	30.144	33.867	36.191	43.820
20	19.337	28.412	31.410	35.020	37.566	45.315
21	20.337	29.615	32.671	36.343	38.932	46.797
22	21.337	30.813	33.924	37.659	40.289	42.268
23	22.337	32.007	35.172	38.968	41.638	49.728
24	23.337	33.196	36.415	40.270	42.980	51.179
25	24.337	34.382	37.652	41.566	44.314	56.620
26	25.336	35.563	38.885	42.856	45.642	54.052
27	26.336	36.741	40.113	44.140	46.963	55.476
28	27.336	37.916	41.337	15.419	48.278	56.893
29	28.336	39.087	42.557	46.693	49.588	58.302
30	29.336	40.256	43.773	47.962	50.892	59.703

Source: Adapted by permission of the authors and publishers from Table IV (Fisher and Yates, 1974).

Table C *Critical values of ϱ (rho) at various levels of probability (Spearman rank correlation coefficient)*

For any *N* the observed value of ρ is significant at a given level of significance if it is *equal* to or *larger* than the critical values shown in the table.

N (number of subjects)	Level of significance for one-tailed test			
	0.05	0.025	0.01	0.005
	Level of significance for two-tailed test			
	0.10	0.05	0.02	0.01
5	0.900	1.000	1.000	–
6	0.829	0.886	0.943	1.000
7	0.714	0.786	0.893	0.929
8	0.643	0.738	0.833	0.881
9	0.600	0.683	0.783	0.833
10	0.564	0.648	0.746	0.794
12	0.506	0.591	0.712	0.777
14	0.456	0.544	0.645	0.715
16	0.425	0.506	0.601	0.665
18	0.399	0.475	0.564	0.625
20	0.377	0.450	0.534	0.591
22	0.359	0.428	0.508	0.562
24	0.343	0.409	0.485	0.537
26	0.329	0.392	0.465	0.515
28	0.317	0.377	0.448	0.496
30	0.306	0.364	0.432	0.478

Note: When there is no exact number of subjects use the next lowest number.

Table D   *Critical values of r at various levels of probability (Pearson product movement correlation)*

For any particular N the observed value of ρ is significant at a given level of significance if it is equal to or larger than the critical values shown in the table.

	Level of significance for one-tailed test				
	0.05	0.025	0.01	0.005	0.005
	Level of significance for two-tailed test				
df=$N-2$	0.10	0.05	0.02	0.01	0.001
1	0.9877	0.9969	0.9995	0.9999	1.0000
2	0.9000	0.9500	0.9800	0.9900	0.9990
3	0.8054	0.8783	0.9343	0.9587	0.9912
4	0.7293	0.8114	0.8822	0.9172	0.9741
5	0.6694	0.7545	0.8329	0.8745	0.9507
6	0.6215	0.7067	0.7887	0.8343	0.9249
7	0.5822	0.6664	0.7498	0.7977	0.8982
8	0.5494	0.6319	0.7155	0.7646	0.8721
9	0.5214	0.6021	0.6851	0.7348	0.8471
10	0.4793	0.5760	0.6581	0.7079	0.8233
11	0.4762	0.5529	0.6339	0.6835	0.8010
12	0.4575	0.5324	0.6120	0.6614	0.7800
13	0.4409	0.5139	0.5923	0.6411	0.7603
14	0.4259	0.4973	0.5742	0.6226	0.7420
15	0.4124	0.4821	0.5577	0.6055	0.7246
16	0.4000	0.4683	0.5425	0.5897	0.7084
17	0.3887	0.4555	0.5285	0.5751	0.6932
18	0.3783	0.4438	0.5155	0.5614	0.6787
19	0.3687	0.4329	0.5034	0.5487	0.6652
20	0.3598	0.4227	0.4921	0.5368	0.6524
25	0.3233	0.3809	0.4451	0.4869	0.5974
30	0.2960	0.3494	0.4093	0.4487	0.5541
35	0.2746	0.3246	0.3810	0.4182	0.5189
40	0.2573	0.3044	0.3578	0.3932	0.4896
45	0.2428	0.2875	0.3384	0.3721	0.4648
50	0.2306	0.2732	0.3218	0.3541	0.4433
60	0.2108	0.2500	0.2948	0.3248	0.4078
70	0.1954	0.2319	0.2737	0.3017	0.3799
80	0.1829	0.2172	0.2565	0.2830	0.3568
90	0.1726	0.2050	0.2422	0.2673	0.3375
100	0.1638	0.1946	0.2301	0.2540	0.3211

Note: When there is no exact df use the next lowest number.

Reference

Fisher, R. and Yates, F. (1974) *Statistical Tables for Biological, Agricultural and Medical Research*. Sixth edition. Longman Group Ltd.

Appendix 4
Construction industry employee injury statistics

A typical example of injuries to employees in the construction industry, as reported to the Health and Safety Executive's Field Operations Division.

Occupation	Fatal	Major	Over 3 days	Total
Bricklayer	2	72	550	624
Carpenter/joiner	2	136	1127	1265
Demolition worker	–	16	37	53
Electrician	–	108	330	438
Glazier	1	12	96	109
Ground worker	4	58	139	201
Painter, decorator	–	61	233	294
Pavior, roadman	3	39	443	485
Pilling hand	1	6	33	40
Plasterer	–	22	158	180
Plumber, pipe fitter	–	71	543	614
Scaffolder	2	62	222	286
Slater, roof worker	7	64	195	266
Steel erector	–	24	36	60
Steel fixer, bar bend	–	10	30	40
Steeplejack	–	6	2	8
Welder	–	20	72	92
Other const. trade	5	109	378	492
Drivers	4	120	539	663
Electrical linesman	–	8	23	31
Electrical fitter	–	10	50	60
Electrical jointer	–	4	14	18
Communications engineer	–	1	8	9
Labourer	9	316	1659	1984
Maintenance personnel	5	60	294	359
All managerial	2	120	473	595
Manual production	2	104	548	654
Other occupations	–	78	623	701
Not known	–	81	520	601
Total	49	1798	9375	11222

Appendix 5
Using SPSS

From Daniel Fong, handout notes to MSc Surveying and Construction Project Management, London South Bank University.

Introduction

SPSS is one of the most widely used statistics analysis packages in providing detailed and comprehensive statistics analysis on various types of data. The spreadsheet-like interface allows users to enter data easily and to conduct in-depth data analysis.

SPSS is often used in research as a tool to analyse survey/questionnaire feedback. Although the graphics output may not have the level of customisation offered by Excel, it is often used in conjunction with Excel to provide full statistical analyses and professional presentation of data in research reports and dissertations.

1. Starting SPSS

Click on **Start** button at bottom left of the screen, then click
All Programs, SPSS Inc, PASW Statistics 18, PASW Statistics 18

The dialog box below will appear:

Check on **Type in data**. The dialog box will disappear and the SPSS Data Editor
will surface.

2.   Data Types

Measurement of Data   **Examples of data**

Non metric data

Nominal	Labels with no mathematical properties such as categories	Profession (Architect, Building Surveyor, Construction Manager). Answer (Yes or No).
Ordinal	Ranked or ordered categories. Difference not in equal proportion	Rank order (1st, 2nd, 3rd, etc.). Academic Qualification (PhD, Masters, Degree, Higher National, A-level equivalent).

Use non-parametric statistical techniques

Metric data

Interval	Ordered in equal interval, with arbitrary zero point	Temperature ($0\,°C \neq$ no temp!). IQ score.
Ratio	Ordered in equal interval, with a real zero	Cost, weight, height.

Use parametric statistical techniques

Discussion: what type of measurement do Likert items conform to:

(Hint: Likert scale of 1–5 typically consists of the following Likert items:)

* Strongly disagree
* Disagree
* Neither agree nor disagree
* Agree
* Strongly agree

3. Data entry

Suppose we send out the following questionnaire to project managers and received 22 responses:

Questionnaire

For the most recent project you have completed, please answer the following questions:

Q1. The original target cost of the project £. . . . .

Q2. The actual cost of the project £. . . . .

Q3. The Health & Safety assessment score (0 – 100) . . . .

The data should be entered in the following way in SPSS with 22 rows, each represents the answers of one responding case:

Question 1   **Question 2**   **Question 3**

	Project	Target	Actual	HS_score	Profit
1	1	346039	295176	90	17
2	2	403450	420000	100	-4
3	3	554950	423863	99	31
4	4	1250000	1098166	100	14
5	5	628000	628000	100	0
6	6	3250000	3050000	96	7
7	7	4152000	2875000	98	44
8	8	1148864	1062446	99	8
9	9	260212	243716	99	7
10	10	1675428	1675428	89	0
11	11	190018	152515	99	25
12	12	6885812	5900000	79	17
13	13	2375012	2300000	96	3
14	14	6000000	3500000	99	71
15	15	2945431	2471812	96	19
16	16	765057	837842	52	-9
17	17	1655476	1701419	70	-3
18	18	449054	445000	81	1
19	19	1675428	1650428	88	2
20	20	2951619	3179997	91	-7
21	21	2350000	1735799	95	35
22	22	221534	191849	98	15

Step 1

The first step is to define the type of data for each column. Switching to **Variable View** allows us to create a structure for the data.

The first data column is Project which is used to label the case.

The second data column refers to the Target cost of the project.

The third data column records the Actual cost of a particular project.

The fourth data column elicits the respective Health & Safety score for the project.

The fifth data column is not from the questionnaire: we define the variable!

* **The Name of a data column must consist of only letters and numbers without any space.** Full text can be entered under **Label**.

Step 2

For this questionnaire, suppose we need to establish an additional fifth column of data which evaluates the profit margin. Click on **Transform**, **Compute Variable** from the menu:

Step 3

Once the structure of all data columns is defined, return to **Data View** to enter the
cases.

	Project	Target	Actual	HS_score	Profit	var	var	var	var
1	1	346039	295176	90	17				
2	2	403450	420000	100	-4				
3	3	554950	423863	99	31				
4	4	1250000	1098166	100	14				
5	5	628000	628000	100	0				
6	6	3250000	3050000	96	7				
7	7	4152000	2875000	98	44				
8	8	1148864	1062446	99	8				
9	9	260212	243716	99	7				
10	10	1675428	1675428	89	0				
11	11	190018	152515	99	25				
12	12	6885812	5900000	79	17				
13	13	2375012	2300000	96	3				
14	14	6000000	3500000	99	71				
15	15	2945431	2471812	96	19				
16	16	765057	837842	52	-9				
17	17	1655476	1701419	70	-3				
18	18	449054	445000	81	1				
19	19	1675428	1650428	88	2				
20	20	2951619	3179997	91	-7				
21	21	2350000	1735799	95	35				
22	22	221534	191849	98	15				

4.   Data analysis

The application of statistics techniques depends on the type of measurement, and what we intend to investigate.

Correlation analysis

Correlation analysis is used to test the hypothesis H_0: **No correlation between variables**

Pearson Coefficient of Correlation is often used to measure if two interval or ratio variables are linearly related. Normality of variables not required. The coefficient r lies between -1 and 1.

* r close to 1   Significant positive relationship between variables
* r close to -1 Significant negative relationship between variables
* r close to 0   Little of no significant relationship

* Note: If the variables are related in a non-linear way, r may have a value close to 0. However, the curvilinear relationship could be uncovered with other statistical techniques. It is therefore recommended to always plot the two variables against each other (scatterplot) and examine any possible relationship visually prior to drawing any conclusion.

To examine if there is any association between H&S Score and Profit, click on **Analyze**, **Correlate**, **Bivariate**. . .

Select and move the two variables to this column

Check **Pearson** correlation coefficient and click OK.

The following results should appear on the **Statistics Viewer**:

A Pearson correlation coefficient r of 0.406 is computed, with a significance of 0.061 (or written as $p = 0.061$).

Normally, a significance of less than 0.05 ($p < 0.05$) is needed to conclude a relationship.

Scatterplot

Go to **Graphs**, **Legacy Dialogs**, **Scatter/Dots . . ., Simple Scatter**

Click **Define**.

Move the two variables under Y and X axes accordingly and click **OK**.

The following chart output will appear.

Although there is no significant linear relationship, a non–linear relationship could be established in this case.

Spearman's rank-order correlation (ρ or r_s) is used to examine if two variables are monotonically associated (both increase at the same time, or one increase and the other increase, not necessary linearly). Both variables must be ordinal or better. Normality of variables is not required.

Although the technique is 'rank-order' based, the data we provide does not have to be. SPSS will process ordinal/interval/ratio data into rank for the analysis.

Click on **Analyze, Correlate, Bivariate** . . . and check box for **Spearman**.

A student conducted a survey to examine the difference in opinion between the size of the firm (1 = small, 2 = medium, 3 = large) in the use of computerised techniques. The question asks for the opinion on whether computer techniques enhance the effectiveness of project management (1 = Strongly agree, 2 = Agree, 3 = Neutral, 4 = Disagree, 5 = Strongly disagree).

```
Spearman.sav [DataSet2] - PASW Statistics Data Editor                    _ |□| X|
File   Edit   View   Data   Transform   Analyze   Graphs   Utilities   Add-ons   Window   Help
```

	Firm	Opinion	var	var	var	var	var
1	1	2					
2	1	5					
3	2	1					
4	3	4					
5	1	3					
6	1	3					
7	2	5					
8	3	1					
9	3	1					
10	3	1					
11	3	1					
12	1	4					
13	1	4					
14	1	4					
15	2	4					

Data View   Variable View

PASW Statistics Processor is ready

RESULTS

Correlations			Firm	Opinion
Spearman's rho	Firm	Correlation Coefficient	1.000	−.529**
		Sig. (2-tailed)	.	.005
		N	26	26
	Opinion	Correlation Coefficient	−.529**	1.000
		Sig. (2-tailed)	0.005	.
		N	26	26

** Correlation is significant at the 0.01 level (2-tailed)

A Spearman's rho of -0.529 is computed with a very high significance of 0.005. Another method to test the strength of relationship between two ordinal (or better) variables is **Kendall's Tau** (τ). It is used to examine if two variables are monotonically associated Normality of variables is not required.

Kendall's Tau b is suitable for square tables and **Kendall's Tau c** is more suited for rectangular tables.

RESULTS

Correlations			H&S score	Percentage of profit
Kendall's tau_b	H&S score	Correlation coefficient	1.000	0.248
		Significance (two-tailed)	.	0.117
		N	22	22
	Percentage of profit	Correlation coefficient	0.248	1.000
		Significance (two-tailed)	0.117	.
		N	22	22

A Kendall's tau b of 0.248 with a significance of 0.117 indicates no relationship between the variables.

REGRESSION

After correlation analysis, suppose a significant linear relation between the two interval/ratio variables is confirmed, we wish to find out **how** the variables are related.

Click on **Analyze**, **Regression**, **Linear** . . .

Question: Which is Dependent and which is Independent and why?

The following results are shown:

Model	Unstandardized Coefficients		Standardized Coefficients	t	Sig.
	B	Std. Error	Beta		
1 (Constant)	−46.328	30.306		−1.529	.0142
H&S score	.652	.328	.406	1.985	0.061

Coefficients[a]

a   Dependent variable: percentage of profit.

In this case, the 'best-fit' line that relates Profit (y) and H&S Score (x) has the equation:

$$y = 0.6546x - 46.328$$

When analysing Nominal variables, Chi-square (χ^2) Test or Fisher's Exact Test is used to compare two groups of data to see if there is a difference between them, or to examine if the variables are related (test of independence).

H_0: No difference between variables

Condition to apply Chi-square test

2-by-2 table	All cells must have a frequency count of at least 5.
Larger tables	80% of the cells have a frequency count of at least 5, and no cell with 0 count.

When the condition is not met, Yates' correction is automatically applied by SPSS.

Condition to apply Fisher's exact test

Small sample, sparse or unbalanced data (<20). No blank cell.
Does not work well when the table is adequately filled.
SPSS automatically generates Fisher's Exact Test results under Chi-square Test when the condition is met.

Suppose we wish to establish if there is a relationship between the size of the firm and its location.

Click on **Analyze, Descriptive Statistics, Crosstabs**. . .

Click **Statistics**.

The following results are shown:

Chi-square tests			
	Value	df	Asymp. Sig. (2-sided)
Pearson chi-square	6.727[a]	8	0.566
Likelihood ratio	8.029	8	0.431
Linear-by-linear association	0.871	1	0.0351
No. of valid cases	26		

a. 15 cells (100.0%) have expected count less than 5. The minimum expected count is 1.08.

This table shows a p of 0.566, which is not significant to reject **H₀**.

For Ordinal variables, **Mann–Whitney U Test (Wilcoxon rank sum W test)** is used to compare two groups of data to see if there is a difference between them. When more than two groups are considered, Kruskal–Wallis One-Way Analysis of Variance (K–W one-way ANOVA or H test) will apply.

It is used when sample sizes are small and/or the variables are not normally distributed. The method can also be used for interval and ratio measurements.

H₀: No difference between variables

For the previous example on examining the difference in opinion between the size of the firm (1=small, 2=medium, 3=large) and on whether computer techniques enhance the effectiveness of project management (1=Strongly agree, 2=Agree, 3 =Neutral, 4=Disagree, 5=Strongly disagree).

Click on **Analyze**, **Nonparametric Tests**, **Independent Samples**. . . and at the following screen, click **Run**:

Move the variables into the corresponding boxes and click Run.

RESULTS

Hypothesis Test Summary

	Null Hypothesis	Test	Sig.	Decision
1	The distribution of Opinion is the same across categories of Firm.	Independent-Samples Kruskal-Wallis Test	.029	Reject the null hypothesis.

Asymptotic significances are displayed. The significance level is .05.

The output from SPSS not only indicates the test it has used but also the decision!

When the measurement is Interval or Ratio, parametric tests are often used. Requirements for Parametric Test:

- Variables must be normally distributed
- Variability of variables should be low (homogeneity of variance)

Parametric methods such as the *t*-Test can be used to test the hypothesis **H₀: no difference between the means of two groups**. In other words, we are testing if there is any difference between the two groups of data.

Suppose we wish compare our research results with those from a previous research.

Click **Analyze**, **Compare Means**, **Independent Samples T Test**. . . Move the variables into the appropriate boxes. You may wish to Define the Groups but it is optional.

Group statistics

	Author	N	Mean	Std. Deviation	Std. Error Mean
Leanness	Taj	65	55.2654	12.29832	1.52542
	Whitwort	37	53.5054	19.81432	3.25745

Independent samples test

		Levene's test for equality of variances		t-test for Equality of Means					95% Confidence Interval of the Difference	
		F	Significance	t	df	Significance (two-tailed)	Mean difference	Standard error of the difference	Lower	Upper
Leanness	Equal variances assumed	16.621	0.000	0.554	100	.581	1.75998	3.17802	-4.54512	8.06508
	Equal variances not assumed			0.489	52.111	.627	1.75998	3.59693	-5.45742	8.97738

To interpret the results, we need to first look under the Levene's test of equality of variances column. $F = 16.6$ is significant ($p = 0.000$) means we have to use the results from the 'Equal variances not assumed' section.

For the results of our *t*-test, a *t*-value of 0.489 at $p = 0.627$ indicates there is no significant difference between the mean leanness score of construction projects surveyed in our research and that of the manufacturing projects in Taj's study.

If we wish to compare more than two means, **One-way ANOVA** is use for interval/ratio data. The conditions to run ANOVA are:

• The groups must be normally distributed.
• The variances of the groups must be equal.

One sample Kolmogorov–Smirnov test is used to check each group of data for normality. If normality does not hold, use the nonparametric **K–W one-way ANOVA** test.

Suppose we wish to examine if there is a difference in productivity between Germany, France, and the UK.

Click **Analyze**, **Compare Means**, **One Way ANOVA**. . . Bring the variables into the right boxes, e.g., Country is the independent factor in this case.

Click **Options** to specify some statistics and a test on equality of variances:

RESULTS

Descriptives								
Productivity								
	N	Mean	Std. Deviation	Std. Error	95% Confidence Interval for Mean		Min.	Max.
					Lower Bound	Upper Bound		
Germany	65	55.2654	12.29832	1.52542	52.2180	58.3128	30.61	77.42
France	37	53.5054	19.81432	3.25745	46.8990	60.1118	11.00	91.60
UK	22	52.7727	20.32810	4.33397	43.7598	61.7857	15.00	90.00
Total	124	54.2980	16.28678	1.46260	51.4029	57.1931	11.00	91.60

df1	df2	Significance
2	121	.000

ANOVA					
Productivity					
	Sum of squares	df	Mean square	F	Significance
Between groups	135.255	2	67.627	0.252	0.778
Within groups	32491.631	121	268.526		
Total	32626.886	123			

In the Descriptives results table, the mean score for the three countries are shown.

As Levene's test of equality of variances shows significant ($p=0.000$) difference between the variances of the three groups, the results of the subsequent ANOVA will not be relied upon in this case.

Appendix 6
Example of presenting interview results in a tabulated format

From an MSc dissertation by Zoë Elizabeth Mulholland (2010, pp. 59–63). The dissertation was supervised by Dr Shamil Naoum, MSc course in Construction Project Management, London South Bank University. For more of this research's findings see Naoum and colleagues (2011).

Question	Client A	Client B	Client C	Architect A	Architect B	Architect C	Cost Manager A	Cost Manager B	Contractor A	Contractor B
Section 2 – Definition										
A) 1. What is your understanding of the term sustainable construction?	Acting responsibly, reducing impact of the company's operations on its surroundings, people and environment.	Briefing/design with renewable; low carbon and low energy 2. Min. waste max prefab. Considerate contractors – no noise or pollution. 3. End product, build quality, longevity and running costs.	Carbon neutrality. The issue of carbon content seems to be driving the sustainable construction. However it is impossible to produce carbon neutral buildings economically.	Holistic view of buildings, thinking about energy, life cycle costs and durability. Not just technology but what you do with the building and how it is operated.	Triple bottom line: Environment; Economy; Society 90% focus on energy/ carbon. But not enough on social side. Get social and environmental aspects right then economics follows.	Totality of the building from the initial concept. Balance between capital cost and running cost. A traditional concept: avoiding waste.	What is developed today can still be developed in future. Minimising the impact on the environment and society. It's not just about being carbon neutral.	Use of renewable resources and materials.	1. Renewable 2. Long term environmental impact.	1. Use of sustainable sources. 2. Design & construction that reduces CO_2.
2. When were you first aware of sustainable construction?	2000 BREEAM was considered. Prior to that thinking about the way we operated e.g. source of timber, how much cement was being used.	2005 Campus consisted of 1960s building not built to last and hard to adapt. Look at Victorian buildings which scrub up really well.	2005/6	Late 1990s, early 2000	Early 1990s	Early 1990s. But more active in the last two years.	2000 Heard about BREEAM	2005/6	2005	2006
Section 3 – Sustainable construction experience										
A) 1. When did you first implement sustainable construction practices?	2001 BREEAM 'Good' rating £65M.	2008 Academic building. New build £60M.	2009 High end residential. PV panels £10M.	2000 Sports centre, £7M BREEAM excellent	1992 Commercial development with displacement vent; retractable shading.	1993 Office with sustainably sourced materials.	2003/4 School project. Rainwater harvesting; low voltage lights; facade performance; landscaping.	2007 Commercial office BREEAM 'Very Good' for operation and maintenance but not design. New build.	2006. Retail project in SE £9M BREEAM 'Very Good'.	2006. Office £7.5M new/part refurbish
2. What sustainable construction practices do you have experience of?	Commercial office. BREEAM 'Excellent' Landmark project in 2009. Waterless urinals; Green roof; Rain water harvesting; Bat boxes; Solar panels covered 30% roof; Bike spaces	Teaching space Medical research Low velocity fume cupboards; Natural ventilation;	Private let new and refurb apartments. Code 4; Ecological & sustainability report; Green roofs; Green walls	Housing association, CfSH L4–6. Office commended for low energy £3.5M using PVs obtain grant funding from DTI. FE College £1M Ground source heat pumps Guesthouse, £1M used biomass boilers.	Further education college 20M 2003 PVs sponsored by the government University admin 20M 2005 PVs 50% grant from the council; external shading BRE house Carbon zero house	HE College new build BREEAM 'Excellent' HE College refurb BREEAM 'Good' Laboratory Bespoke BREEAM	FE College used CHP £20M HEI project energy saving measures FE College BREEAM £20M looked at transport strategies HE College 2007 ground source heat pumps	New build apartments £3.5M 2011 CfSH L4 Supermarket £2.5M 2000 Solar panels; Greywater	Retail £9M 2006 BREEAM 'V.Good' Recycled bottles cladding; Sheep's wool insulation. Bank fit out PIRs; Long life lamps Bank HQ PV panels Retail Grey water; Ground source heat pumps; Green roofs	Office 2006 Energy saving lights Natural ventilation Actuator windows Chimney 'false draught ventilation' Sustainable materials. No technologies used in any of projects.

Question	Client A	Client B	Client C	Architect A	Architect B	Architect C	Cost Manager A	Cost Manager B	Contractor A	Contractor B
Section 4 – Drivers for sustainable construction										
A) In your opinion what are the drivers for sustainable construction?	1. No choice. If you care about the environment got to be done. Think of legacy left for our children. 2. Being 'seen' to be doing good 3. It makes business sense, better ways of doing thing.	1. Funding source, in our case HEFCE, demands it. 2. Reputational issue – hot topic globally. 3. Personal conscience.	1. Planning permission 2. Regulations 3. Customer demand - 20% premium on rent because of the sustainable development demand. 4. Belief that there is an issue that needs to be addressed.	1. Personal agenda of the client 2. Cost of energy. 3. Legislation	1. Funding in the public sector is dependent upon improved sustainability 2. Social benefits 3. Economic, there must be a business case 4. Legislation	1. Funding authority demands it. 2. Legislation 3. Increase in energy cost. 4. Personal commitment to sustainable construction.	1. Public Relations, public perception 2. Energy saving 3. Access to funding	1. Saleability. 2. Ethos of doing green things. 3. Regulations.	1. Image. Seen to be engaging. 2. Personal commitment.	1. Genuine desire to right the wrongs of the past. 2. 'Seen' to be seen to be sustainable. 3. Desire to save on running costs.
B) Rate the importance of these drivers on a scale of 1–10 (where 10 is most important and 1 is not at all).	B) Comment was made and blended within the discussions of the results.	B) Comment	B)	B) Comment	B) Comment	B) Comment	B) Comment	B) Comment	B) Comment	B) Comment
CSR policy	10	7	4	5	3	8	8	6.5	8.5	9
Legislation	5	9	8	7	9	6.5	10	10	10	5
WLC benefits	7.5	7	6	3	Owners – 5 Rent – 1	8.5	5	5	7.5	9
Competitive advantage	10	7	1	5	8	5	3	3	6	1
Customer demand	9	6	6	Public – 7, Private – 3	6	5	Public 10 Private 8	2	9.5	8
Green incentives	7	6	3	9	8	7	6	6	2	6
Peer pressure	2	9	3	6	4	4.5	8	4	8	9
Better buildings	10	8	7	6	7	8.5	7	2	7	6

C) In light of the recession, do you think these drivers will increase (I), decrease (D) or not change (NC)?	C)	Comment	C)	Comment	C)	Comment	C)	Comment	C)	Comment	C)	Comment	C)	Comment	C)	Comment	C)	Comment	C)	Comment
CSR policy	NC		D		D	More concerned about bottom line	NC		NC		NC		NC		NC		I		D	
Legislation	NC		D		I	Legislation is going to increase	I		NC		I	New Part L even more onerous.	I		NC		NC		NC	
WLC benefits	NC		D	Clients focus on the initial capital costs	I	Oil more expensive plus increasing energy demand	I		D	Clients do not see beyond the initial outlay	I		NC		I	Benefit realised of lower running costs	I	Running costs will increase	I	Clients focus on running costs.
Competitive advantage	I	Bigger incentive to differentiate your business	I	Need to distinguish themselves	NC		NC		I	Need to be more competitive in recession	NC		I		I	Do anything to distinguish yourself from competition	I	Desperate for anything to give an advantage	I	Do anything to increase advantage
Customer demand	I		NC		I	As awareness grows so will demand	I, D	Public – increase Private – decrease	I		I	Customers are gradually becoming more aware	I, NC	Public – increase Private – no change	NC		I		NC	Depends on the client and project.
Green incentives	NC		D	Less money around, even from Gov.	I	Green bank noted in Gov. 2010 budget	NC		I		I	Follow from legislation.	D		I		NC	But note 9 for Education more grants	NC	
Peer pressure	NC		NC		D		D		NC		NC		NC		NC		NC		NC	
Better buildings	I		D	A nice to have not essential.	NC		D		D	Clients cannot afford these measures	I		I		NC		I	Best possible for least amount	NC	

Section 5 – *Barriers to sustainable construction*

Question	Client A	Client B	Client C	Architect A	Architect B	Architect C	Cost Manager A	Cost Manager B	Contractor A	Contractor B
A) In your opinion what are the barriers to sustainable construction?	People do not like change.	1. Larger capital outlay. 2. Difficult to persuade academics of the importance. 3. End users are very intolerant of change.	1. Technology not as advanced as the politicians state, 2. Lack of transparency of the feed-in tariffs/ grants. 3. Building industry set in their ways.	1. Lack of knowledge of the benefits. 2. Reluctant to change way of working. 3. Limit of technology –no track record 4. Perception of cost.	1. Not enough in-use and capital cost data. 2. Cost 3. Changing legislation. 4. Risk of emerging technology.	1. Perception that it costs more money. 2. Split incentives.	1. Public perception: unaffordable and does not work, 2. "eco bling", BREEAM just a badge. 3. Difficult to refurb existing buildings.	1. Capital cost. 2. Non standard installations. 3. Perception that it is more expensive to run.	1. Clients do not know what is out there and are unfamiliar. 2. Resistance to change. 3. Perception of cost.	1. Increased capital outlay. 2. Lack true desire and interest 3. Too risky in a recession 4. Poor professional advice. 5 CDM – access and maintenance can be costly.
B) Rate the importance of these barriers on a scale of 1–10.	B) Comment	B) Comment	B) Comment	B) Comment	B) Comment	B) Comment	B) Comment	B) Comment	B) Comments	B) Comments
Increased capital outlay	5 — If thought about early enough then no increase.	10	8	8	8	8	10	8	7	8
Lack of demand	2 — Huge demand, customers need to be seen to be green.	3	5	8	6	8	8	9	6	7
Physical barriers	5	8	8	5	5	8	8	8	6	8
Poor knowledge by client	1 — Developer has their own sustainability department	3	7	8	6	3	7	9	3	8
Split incentive	7 — Need to educate the client	4	8	8	8	6	10	8	7	9
Unknowns of new tech	5 — Need more new tech; old products and ideas	8	9	8	7	3	7	5	5	5
SME	2	7	5	7	4	8	8	7	7	7
Lack of training	4	3	3	3	5	7	3	5	3	4

C) In light of the recession, do you think these drivers will increase (I), decrease (D) or not change (NC)?	C)	Comment	C)	Comment	C)	Comment	C)	Comment	C)	Comment	C)	Comment	C)	Comments	C)	Comments
Increased capital outlay	I	Clients focus on every penny of expenditure	NC		D	As tech and competition improves capital costs will go down.	I		D	Clients see as an opportunity for saving money.	I		I		I	
Lack of demand	NC		D	Increased awareness and changing attitudes	D	Increasing awareness and growing demand	I		D	There will be an increase in demand.	I		I	People are just not spending.	NC	
Physical barriers	I		D	Industry find new ways of working and adapt	NC		NC		D	Greater application of sustainable construction in all areas.	NC	There will have to be more refurb	D		NC	
Poor knowledge by client	D	Projects on hold there so more time to explore.	D		NC		NC		NC		NC		NC	Education and but not commercial	NC	
Split incentive	D	Tenants are trying to be more efficient with current financial pressures.	NC		NC		NC		D	More holistic approach will be taken due to the economic situation.	NC		I		I	Pressure on capital budgets not FM
Unknowns of new tech	NC		D		D	We will become more familiar with the technology	NC		D	Increasing awareness and benefits of new technologies realised.	I		I		NC	
SME	I		NC		I	SMEs cannot access debt, let alone pay premium for sustainability	NC		D		NC	No change to those with small portfolio	I		NC	
Lack of training	NC		D		D	As with awareness it is improving	I	Reduced training with budgets cuts	D		NC		I	Very diverse among sector	NC	

Question	Client A	Client B	Client C	Architect A	Architect B	Architect C	Cost Manager A	Cost Manager B	Contractor A	Contractor B
A)1. In what ways has your organisation been affected by the recession?	All work on hold. Last development came to the market in 2009. The next development is likely to be in 2011.	Moderate effect. Cut in capital spend 10% voluntary redundancy. But science is well supported by the government.	Moderate effect. All building is focused on rent income. Rent reduced by 7–8%. There is a much higher risk of contractors going bust.	Moderate, Maybe in future. Large number of bids but projects are not being commissioned. Ones that are – smaller budgets, lower fees.		Moderate effect.	Moderate but boosted by public work. Fewer project with smaller budgets. Increased competition for work. Redundancies.	Moderate. Starting to notice downturn in projects as public sector slowing down. Staff redundancies.	Smaller value projects; more tendering opportunities but with bigger list; reduced margins and some negative bids. Projects awarded but on hold.	Reduce turnover and costs. Stiffer competition. Larger contractors are dropping down to smaller works as there are less big projects.
2. Which industry or clients have been worst affected?	Commercial office	Housing	Residential	Commercial office			Commercial	HE	Commercial dried up	Financial
B)1. Since the recession have you encountered a change in the amount of sustainable construction?	Yes, increase.	Increase. Only just started in past two years.	Increase	No change	Decrease	Increase. Sustainability become higher profile.	Increase because of legislation	No change.		It's being talked about less, finding it is less of a driver.
2. Since the recession has there been a change in the type of sustainable construction?	Yes, in future going to really challenge approach to building. Buildings will be dramatically different. Look at air flow, orientation, shading – focus on passive measures.	Considered using PVs but removed because of their poor WLC not because of the recession – even if the project budget was more flexible it would not have been implemented.	CfSH reduced from L6 to L4 to make a viable return. Future is domestic CHP cheap electricity and potential income from feed-in tariffs up to 40% reduction in running costs. Passive measure, i.e. insulation. Project completed in 2009 full of air conditioning – never again. Market will accept natural ventilation.	More emphasis on passive approach by using efficient materials and design. PVs are excluded from projects unless they are subsidised by some form of grant. Code 6 housing has increased		More formal measures being used like BREEAM. About achieving targets rather than talking about it. SWMP legislation is proof.	PVs and other renewable energy tech were used before. Now rationalising existing stock. BREEAM will continue to be used a "stamp" of sustainability. More refurbishment rather than new build.	Level to which they are implemented has sometimes be downgraded. E.g. pipeline development is going from Code 6 to 4 due to financial constraints. Hospital new build project still going for BREEAM excellent.	Awareness increased. More focus on natural ventilation. Increased number of suppliers providing renewable technologies and the competition is increasing among them. Lack of new ideas. Always natural ventilation; rainwater harvesting; green roof Need more innovation	Small/medium jobs do not address sustainable construction in a major way. Only minor details such as PIRs etc not bigger investments like technologies.

3. In your opinion what is the cause for these changes?	Using two year gap to innovate. Tenants are being educated; they will accept wider temperature ranges.	As we are really looking to save money the focus is on air conditioning as it has potential to be a huge saving if removed. Need strong business case and energy efficiency provides that. Convenient that this is being 'green'.	Running costs and capital. Air conditioning very expensive. People are aware enough of the environmental issues to put up with warmer environments.	Running costs need to be reduced in future. Otherwise need Government grant in order to subsidise other renewable technologies.	Increased pressure on capital budgets, opportunity to invest decreases. Each project is subject to much great scrutiny. The 2%, 5%, 10% increase for sustainable buildings is not justifiable.	Organisations are concerned about energy efficiency, material and maintenance. The recession will not make people go backwards legislation will ensure that.	Lack of capital funding. Running costs of building for owner/occupiers.	Clients better educated but also they are looking to save money. Clients are switched on about saving on maintenance costs. No longer blinkered.
4. Which sectors do you think have been the most willing to continue with sustainable construction?	All.	Higher Education	Institutions education; hospitals; local government; prime residential. Green leases will push the commercial world longer term.	Social housing; Higher Education. This is where funding is still available.	Education and any other sector where their funding source stipulates sustainable buildings	All of the public related sectors.	Public as the sustainable construction agenda is driven by central government. Legally binding commitments to reduce CO_2.	Good intentions but companies just want to look good. Most initiatives government led – legislation or incentives. Contractors only have a minor role limited to construction phase.

Note to students: The above table should be inserted at the start of the results chapter and each section should be analysed and discussed individually. For example, Zoë analysed and discussed the sections on the definition of sustainability and the barriers to sustainability (as seen by the interviewees) as follows:

Definition of sustainable construction

A broad range of responses were given for the definition of sustainable construction. Some respondents gave very specific responses such as 'being carbon neutral' while other detailed more in depth definitions touching some of the complexities of the field. In particular, Client B gave a detailed outline of what it means from design, construction to occupation of a building. Nevertheless, there were common themes with many overlapping definitions. The most common statements were: to reduce the impact of construction on people and the environment; a holistic approach to building and; the use of renewable energy and materials. It is interesting to note that both the Contractors responses focused on renewable energy and materials as this is the end of the supply chain with which they are involved. The more general concepts of holistic buildings and impact on society or surrounding environment are mentioned by architects and clients. Client B also mentioned under the broader definition of sustainability that the 'Considerate Contractors' Scheme' was key with its bid to reduce impact of noise and prevent pollution to the surrounding area during the construction of a building.

The next most common definitions were low or zero carbon status buildings and consideration of life cycle costing and running costs. Finally, minimising waste in design and construction and longevity of buildings were stated by two of the interviewees. It was noted by Architect C that these last two concepts were in fact very old fashion ideas and stated that 100 years ago all construction professionals were interested in building to last and reducing costly waste.

Some respondents also stated what they considered not to be sustainable construction. Cost Manager A and Architect B made the point that it is not just about being carbon neutral but must be a more far sighted view of the impact on the society and environment. Similarly, Architect A asserts that sustainable construction is not just about technology but how buildings are used and operated.

The wide ranging answers showed that there was a good body of knowledge amongst the respondents, with many demonstrating a deep level of understanding.

An interesting trend can be seen in the timeline of when respondents became aware of sustainable construction (Figure A6.1). Two of the architects had heard of the concept of sustainable construction under different terminology in the early 1990s. These concepts have been dubbed 'proto sustainability' and include energy saving, ethically resourced materials and non polluting construction. In the late 1990s a second group (a client, the other architect and a cost manager working

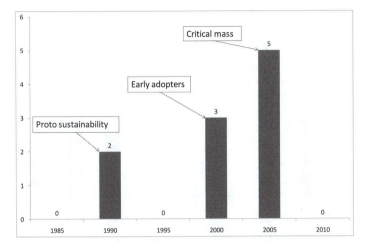

Figure A6.1 *Timeline showing frequency of when respondents first heard about sustainable construction.*

at a dynamic practice) were introduced to the concept. These probably represent 'early adopters' of sustainable construction in its current format, working on landmark projects, first examples of BREEAM and with forward thinking clients. Then there is the critical mass, where half of the other interviewees stated that they had first heard about it in 2005 or 2006. Both contractors state this as the time they became aware of sustainable construction.

Drivers for sustainable construction

The first part, investigating the drivers for sustainable construction, asked respondents to give their opinion on the top drivers without prompting from a list to exclude any bias from academic literature. This gives an overview of their perception from personal or company experience of the subject matter. There was a danger that interviewees could state what they felt they ought to but they were encouraged to be candid in their responses.

The open ended responses were coded into eight categories, which were then grouped in three themes: social, financial and external drivers. Figure A6.2 shows the results according to the frequency with which each driver was mentioned. By a clear margin the most frequent answer was personal commitment of the client or developer with 80 per cent of respondents stating this was a key driver. The next highest at 50 per cent were reputation/image and funding/planning authority demands. These were closely followed by legislation and increased energy costs at 40 per cent. It is worthy of note that only two of the ten respondents stated business case or customer demand as a motivation for adopting sustainable construction, areas which traditionally would be considered a strong driving force behind company strategies.

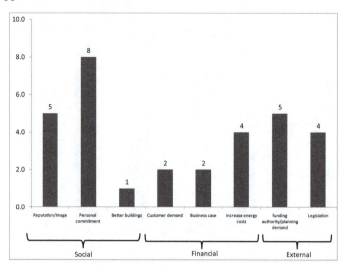

Figure A6.2 *Frequency of drivers for sustainable construction stated unprompted by respondents.*

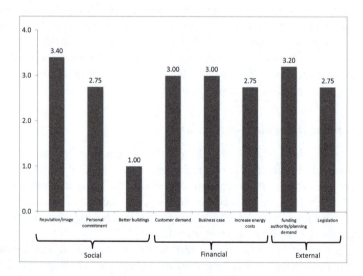

Figure A6.3 *Drivers for sustainable construction with priority ranking stated by respondents unprompted. The higher the bar, the more often the driver was stated first by respondents (the scale has arbitrary units).*

When the results are weighted according to the order in which the respondents listed the drivers a different trend appears (the first response was assumed to be the most important for the respondent, the second assumed to be the second most important, and so on). Figure A6.3 reveals that a company's concern for their reputation or image overtakes personal commitment to be the top priority, showing that the clients in the construction industry are primarily concerned with being 'seen to be green'. Closely behind reputational drivers is the external demand of the funding/planning authority. The two respondents that did state customer demand and business case as drivers for sustainable development ranked them very highly raising their profile in the results. With such a small sample size, single or infrequently listed drivers can distort the results. However it is worth noting that there is a group of respondents that not only consider customer demand and business case as a driver for sustainability but rate it as a top priority.

Reference

Mulholland, Z.E. (2010) 'An examination of sustainable construction in the recession', MSc dissertation, Department of the Built Environment, London South Bank University.

Naoum, S., Mulholland, Z., Fong, D. (2011)'Sustainable Construction in the Recession'. 11th World Sustainable Building Conference SB11, October, Helsinki, Finland. Paper ID 1666853.

Appendix 7
Scoring matrix of project performance

Source: Naoum, S. (1989) 'An investigation into the performance of management contracts and the traditional methods of building procurement', PhD thesis, Brunel University, Middlesex.

Notes to students:

1 This is an example of an achieved research aim. The aim of this research was to construct a scoring matrix showing the level of performance between management and traditional form of contracts (see proposal 2 in Appendix 1).
2 This scoring matrix is related to the research road map shown in Figure 9.2 on p. 130 and also to the research model shown in Figure 9.3 on p. 134.
3 This type of an achieved aim (i.e end of research product) is usually inserted in the conclusion chapter of your dissertation.
4 The content of this scoring matrix may not apply to today's clients' and projects' criteria as the characteristics of the construction industry have changed significantly over the last two decades or so.

Client and project characteristics	Project performance																					
	Management contracts											Traditional contracts										
	Design time	Build time	Total time	Speed (a/w)	Unit cost	% ±time	% +/- cost	Level S time	Level S cost	Level S quality	Total scores	Design time	Build time	Total time	Speed (a/w)	Unit cost	% +/- time	% +/- cost	Level S time	Level S cost	Level S quality	Total scores
Speculative<£5m N=4MC. 3 TR	2	1	2	1	2	1	2	2	2	2	17	1	2	1	3	3	2	2	3	3	3	23
Speculative>£5m N=14MC. 6TRC	3	2	3	3	1	2	3	2	2	1	22	2	2	2	3	3	2	2	3	2	3	24
Bespoke<£5m N=12MC. 11TRC	3	2	3	3	1	2	2	3	3	3	25	1	2	2	2	3	2	2	2	3	2	21
Bespoke>£5m N=7MC. 4TRC	3	2	3	3	3	2	2	3	3	2	26	2	1	1	3	2	2	3	2	2	2	20
Bid rate<50,000 N=10MC. 21 TRC	3	2	2	2	1	3	3	3	3	2	24	2	2	1	3	3	2	2	2	2	3	21
Bid rate>50,000 N=29MC. 9TRC	3	2	3	3	1	3	2	2	3	2	24	1	2	1	1	2	1	1	1	3	2	17
Industrial<£5m N=8MC. 13TRC	3	2	3	3	2	3	2	2	3	3	26	2	2	2	3	3	3	1	2	3	3	22
Industrial>£5m N=8MC. 5TRC	3	2	3	3	3	3	2	23	3	3	27	1	2	1	2	3	1	2	2	2	3	20
Commercial<£5m N=8MC. 5TRC	3	1	3	2	1	3	2	3	2	2	22	2	2	2	3	3	2	3	3	2	3	25
Commercial>£5m N=18MC. 8TRC	3	2	3	2	1	3	2	3	3	2	24	1	1	1	3	2	2	1	1	2	3	17
Area<7000 sqm N=15MC. 18TRC	3	3	3	2	1	2	3	3	2	2	24	2	2	2	2	2	2	2	3	3	3	24
Area>7000 sqm N=24MC. 12TRC	3	2	3	3	3	3	2	3	2	2	28	1	2	1	3	2	2	2	2	2	3	20
Normal complexity N=20MC. 20TRC	3	2	3	2	2	3	3	3	2	2	26	1	2	1	2	3	2	1	2	2	3	19
Highly complex N=19MC. 8TRC	3	2	3	3	2	2	2	3	2	1	23	1	1	1	3	3	2	1	1	2	2	17
TOTALS	44	29	43	37	26	36	34	39	39	31	358	22	26	21	35	41	31	27	31	40	41	315

Measurements

Average performance for projects costing less than £5 million: design time=34 weeks; building time=52 weeks; total time=96 weeks; speed (a/w) =81 area/week; cost/sqm=562 £/sqm; % ± time=5%; % ± time=5%

Average performance for projects costing more than £5 million: design time=55 weeks; building time=88 weeks; total time=140 weeks; speed (a/w) =125 sqm/week; cost/sqm=775 £/sqm; % +/- time=8%; % ± time=7%

Score 1=low performance; score 2=average performance; score 3=high performance.

Index

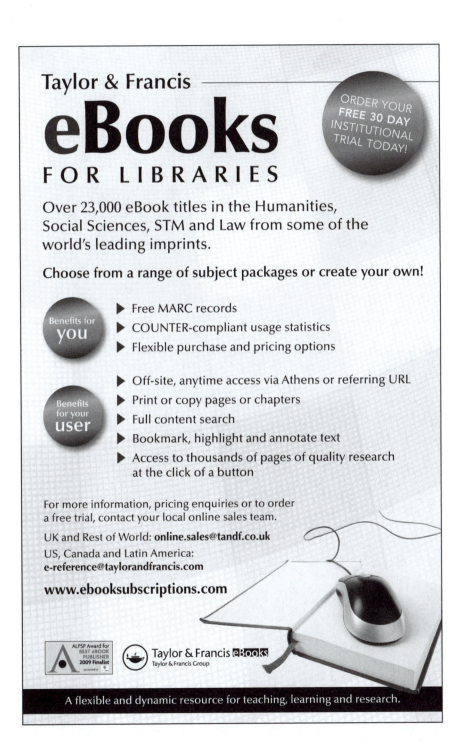